Atlas of Major Thoracoscopic Pediatric Lung Resection for Congenital Pulmonary Airway Malformation

Arnaud Bonnard

Atlas of Major Thoracoscopic Pediatric Lung Resection for Congenital Pulmonary Airway Malformation

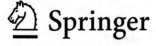

Arnaud Bonnard
Robert Debre Children Univ. Hospital
Paris, France

ISBN 978-3-031-07939-9   ISBN 978-3-031-07937-5   (eBook)
https://doi.org/10.1007/978-3-031-07937-5

This Springer imprint is published by the registered company Springer Nature Switzerland AG
The registered company address is: Gewerbestrasse 11, 6330 Cham, Switzerland

Foreword

Over the last 30 years minimally invasive surgery has taken an ever-expanding and important role in pediatric surgery. Not only does it decrease the pain, scaring, and recovery associated with any given operation, but it minimizes the long-term morbidity associated with these procedures. This is especially important in thoracic surgery in infants and children where it is known that an open thoracotomy is associated with a high degree of chest wall deformity, scoliosis, and muscle girdle weakness. One of our major tasks as pediatric surgeons must be to decrease or eliminate the surgical consequences of our incisions for the benefit of our patients.

Perhaps no procedure offers more of a challenge and creates more angst in the heart of pediatric surgeons than performing complex lung surgery, especially lobectomies. The concerns are many and involve anesthetic issues, a lack of volume of these cases and thus comfort with the anatomy and techniques involved, and the real possibility of major bleeding from the pulmonary vessels. For this reason, I have spent much of my career trying to develop techniques, instruments, and learning tools to help other surgeons overcome these obstacles.

In 2016 I had the great honor of having Arnaud Bonnard come to Denver with his family for a 6-month observership. That time allowed me to come to know him as a great friend, fellow adventurer, and surgical pioneer. Since then, he has clearly distinguished himself as one of the leading MIS surgeons in Europe, and one of the top thoracoscopists in the world.

This Atlas is a gift from Arnaud to all pediatric surgeons who wish to perform thoracoscopic lobectomy. It is a detailed and well-thought-out guide to thoracoscopic lobectomy. His step-by-step approach and illustrations will help with understanding the anatomy, the techniques required, and the preoperative and postoperative care for patients undergoing thoracoscopic lobectomy. While there are always some mild variations between surgeons, Arnaud's in-depth descriptions, illustrations, and thoughtful approach will aid all surgeons attempting these complex and difficult procedures.

Rocky Mountains Children Hospital   Steven Rothenberg
Denver, Colorado, USA

Warning

This manuscript reports a major pulmonary resection technique in children but does not intend to replace all the other techniques described and used by other surgeons. A work of standardization and homogeneity of the technique was developed for the different resections in order to introduce automatisms for the operator, allowing to repeat the procedures and to be able to adapt in the occurrence of peroperative complications. The techniques described make it possible to overcome difficulties related to the anatomy itself and allow a reproducible gesture, in complete safety.

The videos you will be able to watch have been mostly recorded during procedures performed by a fellow or a senior surgeon in the process of acquiring the technique, in order to show that this technique can be easily transmitted and is reproducible. Please note that these videos are speechless showing only the procedure without any comment or image stop.

The techniques described are performed by exclusive thoracoscopy, without assistance by mini-thoracotomy as described in adults by some authors.

Preface

There are surgeries of which one makes a mountain... it is by succeeding for the first time in your career that you can realize that the mountain was actually a molehill. To climb a mountain, you need performant equipment and instruments, tips that you will have gleaned from the sandstone of your career, and, of course, good physical condition but which we will not talk about in this book.

I acquired the tips by observing and working with the pioneers of minimally invasive pediatric surgery. In 2006, when I arrived in Toronto to do a fellowship in neonatal surgery at the Hospital for Sick Children, I still lacked the tricks to be able to perform thoracoscopic lung surgery. Thanks to my mentor, Professor de Lagausie, I had already acquired solid foundations in minimally invasive surgery from the beginning of the 2000s. However, some elements were still missing to be able to treat pulmonary malformations using a thoracoscopic approach in a safe and repro-ducible way. Looking back, I can now identify what I lacked: audacity, a bit of luck, and a book that described a surgical technique making this procedure reproducible and reliable. Back from Toronto, I performed my first thoracoscopic lobectomy, which was an upper right lobectomy. Thanks to Peter Kim and Jack Langer, who gave me the audacity to start ... I never stopped. Over the years, by accumulating crucial details, this procedure has become simple, reproducible, and most impor-tantly successful in avoiding conversion to open surgery.

This book was designed to provide all the tools and steps necessary to success-fully perform thoracoscopic lung resections in children. I do not claim to replace this technique and procedure with another. I simply claim that this technique works and will give you the keys to making thoracoscopic lung resection a relatively sim-ple surgery. The positioning of the patient, surgeon, and laparoscopic column, as well as the trocar placement are identical, regardless of the location of the lesion to resect. Difficulties you may be encountered during the procedure are discussed, as well as solutions to overcome them. Postoperative consequences and complications and their management are also reviewed. The different surgical stages of each lobectomy are supported by numerous photos, anatomical pictures, and videos. Some may already be old, but it is hoped for a second edition with higher and improved quality videos. The instruments used remain 5-mm, although 3-mm instruments have now been developed to perform this surgery. These 3-mm instruments are unfortunately not available in all centers, which is why I believe it is crucial to initially perform and master the technique with 5-mm instruments.

Finally, I would like to thank Dr. Steve Rothenberg. I had the chance to spend 7 months at Rocky Children Hospital in Denver. He is an exceptional and outstanding surgeon and gave me the honor of writing the foreword to this book. He has also helped me improve the thoracoscopic lung surgery technique described in this book, by developing the 5-mm endo-stapler.

I hope this book will meet the readers' expectations. It is one of a kind and I aimed to provide them with exactly the book that I wished I had when I began practicing thoracoscopic lung surgery. Happy reading and re-reading!

Paris, France   Arnaud Bonnard

Acknowledgments

Since 2007, pulmonary resections in children have been performed at Robert-Debré University Hospital by thoracoscopy. This would not have been possible without Prof. El Ghoneimi, head of the Department of Pediatric Digestive, Thoracic, and Urology Surgery, who has always been a support for the development of innovative surgery in his department. In addition, I want to thank the people in the operating room. Each and every one has participated in the development of this technique which has now become a routine procedure at Robert-Debré University Hospital. Of course, without the help of the anesthesiologists with specific techniques required during surgery and especially the contribution and progress of postoperative analgesia, this surgery could not have been performed and the concept of early rehabilitation and enhanced recovery would not have been introduced.

At last, I would like to thank Dr. Louise Montalva who has been working with us since November 2020 as a fellow in our department. She is subspecializing in thoracic, digestive, and neonatal surgery. She has been kind to review this book and its translation in English.

Contents

1 **Pediatric Considerations and Anatomy** 1
   1.1 Introduction. 1
   1.2 The Timing of the Surgery 2
   1.3 Anatomy and Variations to Consider Before Thoracoscopic
       Pulmonary Resections. 3
   References. 9

2 **Technical Considerations and Postoperative Analgesia** 11
   2.1 Patient Positioning, Preparation, and Room Setup 11
   2.2 Instrumentation 13
       2.2.1 Thoracoscopy Instruments 13
       2.2.2 Hemostasis Instruments 16
       2.2.3 Mechanical Stapler. 17
       2.2.4 Endobag 18
   2.3 Placement and Positioning of the Trocars. 18
   2.4 Vascular Control: Bleeding Management 19
   2.5 Bronchial Control: Management of Air Leaks 20
   2.6 Drainage 21
   References. 22

3 **"Tips and Tricks" and Management of Peroperative Difficulties
   and Complications** 23
   3.1 I Need to Ventilate because the Child Is Desaturating 23
   3.2 I Have No Space to Work 24
   3.3 My Fissure Is Complete 24
   3.4 It Is Bleeding and I Cannot See. 25
   3.5 I Cannot Find My Artery. 26
   3.6 I Don't Recognize the Anatomy 26
   3.7 I Cannot Find My Minor Fissure. 26
   3.8 My Remaining Lobe Is Not Ventilating Well 26
   Reference 27

**4   Postoperative Management: Chest-X-Ray—Management of
      Complications and Postoperative Pain—Follow-Up** 29
      4.1 Postoperative Chest X-Ray 29
      4.2 Immediate Complications (Recovery Room) 30
           4.2.1 Bubbling in the Chest Tube 30
           4.2.2 Bleeding or Oozing of Postoperative Secretions
                  Through the Openings of the Trocars. 30
           4.2.3 Subcutaneous Emphysema (Clinical and Radiological). 30
           4.2.4 Accidental Removal of the Nasogastric Tube 30
           4.2.5 Postoperative Pneumothorax (PNO). 31
      4.3 Complications During the Hospital Stay. 31
           4.3.1 Persistent Bubbling. 31
           4.3.2 Persistent Pneumothorax Despite Drainage 31
           4.3.3 Bloody Drainage. 32
      4.4 Pain Management 33
      4.5 Follow-Up 33
      References. 34

5   Lobectomies. 35
      5.1 Upper Lobectomy 35
           5.1.1 Right Upper Lobectomy. 36
           5.1.2 Left Upper Lobectomy 44
      5.2 Middle Lobectomy 50
           5.2.1 Anatomic Findings 50
           5.2.2 First Step: Controlling the Inferior Root of the
                  Superior Pulmonary Vein 51
           5.2.3 Second Step: The Middle Lobe Bronchus
                  or the Medial Artery 53
           5.2.4 Third Step: Controlling the Lateral Artery 54
           5.2.5 Fourth Step: Completing the Fissure 55
           5.2.6 Lower Lobectomy. 56
           5.2.7 Right Lower Lobectomy. 56
           5.2.8 Left Lower Lobectomy. 66
      Further Reading 72

6   Segmentectomy 73
      6.1 Anatomical Segmentectomy 73
           6.1.1 Prerequisite: A 3D Imaging Planner. 73
           6.1.2 Isolating the Artery with an Antegrade Dissection. 75
           6.1.3 Controlling the Segmental Bronchus 79
           6.1.4 Sectioning the Vein. 83
           6.1.5 Sectioning the Parenchyma 83
      Further Reading 84

Conclusion 85

Pediatric Considerations and Anatomy

1

1.1 Introduction

The establishment of a thoracoscopic surgery program in children, and in particular regarding congenital pulmonary malformations (CPAM), must be considered early, well before the first eligible patients. It is necessary to study, for example, the number of patients that this can represent. Indeed, if it speaks to little more than one patient per year, it does not have to be. On the other hand, we must be able to integrate the fact that such a program can allow the development of minimally invasive thoracic surgery in the broad sense by including other malformations such as digestive duplications, bronchogenic cysts, and even surgery for aortic malformations. However, surgery for pulmonary malformations must of course be performed safely and requires advanced training. This training can be done through organized teaching (university courses, specific conference courses, IRCAD), by learning from a colleague, by fellowships or observerships, abroad, or in another department.

In addition, the implementation of such a program cannot be done without the establishment of a close collaboration with the anesthesia team on one hand, and the operating room (OR) team on the other hand. Indeed, everything should not be stammered but thought before. From the installation, through the preparation of the child, to the anesthesia, all this sequence must become "a routine," which is the only guarantee of optimal safety. The "check-list" must obviously be carried out, but most of all, the surgeon must meticulously verify all the prepared instruments, the forceps, and coagulation systems, and must check the parameters of the laparoscopy column with the OR nurse.

In Europe, only half of the pediatric surgeons consider thoracoscopy for surgical treatment of lung malformations [1]. This can be in part explained by the small volume of malformations to be operated on, which makes it difficult to learn the

A. Bonnard, *Atlas of Major Thoracoscopic Pediatric Lung Resection for Congenital Pulmonary Airway Malformation*, https://doi.org/10.1007/978-3-031-07937-5_1

technique and make it reproducible. The aim of this atlas is therefore to help over-come this difficulty.

This atlas will not talk about the combined open-thoracoscopic approach which can nevertheless be an intermediate step between the exclusively open and the exclusively minimally invasive approach. In fact, exposure can be facili-tated by making a 5–6 cm incision, if necessary, with the help of an Alexis retractor [2]. However, this technique requires a learning curve, a thoracotomy incision, and thus joins the criticisms that can be made with fully open techniques.

1.2   The Timing of the Surgery

The timing of surgery has often been a matter of debate. Many people still believe that the older the child, the easier the surgery. Although I would like to be able to show them otherwise, such evidence is lacking in the published literature. The two main arguments for early surgery are the occurrence of complications related to these malformations, such as infections, which is significant in the first years of life (up to 34% of the children develop symptoms of infection during the first year of life as published by Khosa et al. in 2004) [3] and increased lung overgrowth after resection in the young child [4]. In addition, anatomic fissures are often complete in infants, which facilitates the dissection, and postoperative recovery is improved. In our institution's cohort of patients, the decrease in the age at surgery over the last decade from 9 months to 4 months did not modify postoperative morbidity and even allowed the development of enhanced recovery after surgery, with early reha-bilitation [5]. However, Langer et al. recently reported the absence of difference in terms of respiratory function between patients operated on early (3 days) or later (56 months) [4]. However, bias in this latter study might be related to the surgical approach used, as a thoracotomy in 1985 certainly does not have the same impact on growth as a thoracoscopy in 2002. Finally, Boubnova et al. reported no differ-ence in terms of length of hospitalization, duration of drainage, and rate of postop-erative complications between a population of children operated on before 6 months after 6 months [6]. In addition, nowadays, more than 90% of pulmonary malformations are diagnosed prenatally. In fact, it can already be sometimes diffi-cult to explain to parents the presence of a lesion at risk of developing complica-tions that will be managed expectantly during the first months of life.

For these reasons, we recommend early surgery, as early as the third month of age (it is even performed earlier by some authors). A CT scan is performed between 1 and 3 months of age, and often offers high-quality images, with the rapid acquisi-tions of recent CTs, in a sleeping infant [7]. This usually allows the identification of the lesion, its location within a segment, one or several lobes, as well as the possible coexistence of a malformation such as a sequestration with a cystic lesion. Performing a CT scan between 1 and 3 months of age allows accurate surgical plan-ning. This atlas will not discuss the well-debated indication of lobectomy vs conser-vative segmentectomy. Our main focus will be major lobectomies, with a short section on segmentectomy techniques.

1.3   Anatomy and Variations to Consider Before Thoracoscopic Pulmonary Resections

Pulmonary anatomy should be well known before considering a pulmonary resection. Indeed, surgical planification is mandatory and many anatomical landmarks should be identified before surgery. A 3D CT scan reconstruction (3D modeling) can be used to help the surgeon. It can be especially useful for sparing surgery for bilateral lesions or multiple locations within a lung. Even for lobectomies, 3D modeling can facilitate the surgery by showing the number and location of the arteries that need to be controlled. Indeed, anatomic variations are numerous in lung and 3D modeling can be very helpful for the surgeon. A solution like Visible Patient (and the software VP Planning), distributed by Ethicon Johnson and Johnson (France, Issy-les-Moulineaux), is one the best tools for such preoperative planning [8].

As detailed below for each lobectomy, the right lung has 3 lobes, divided in 10 segments, 3 in the right upper lobe, 2 in the middle lobe, and 5 in the right lower lobe. The left lung has 2 lobes, each divided in 5 segments. The superior left lobe contains the culmen (3 segments) and the lingula (2 segments). Each segment receives a main bronchus (B1 to B10—Figs. 1.1, 1.2 and 1.3), artery (A1 to A10—Figs. 1.4 and 1.5), and vein (V1 to V10—Figs. 1.6 and 1.7).

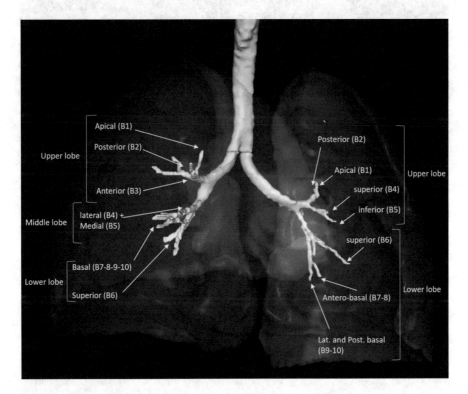

Fig. 1.1 Anatomy of the bronchi—frontal view (Visible Patient™ software)

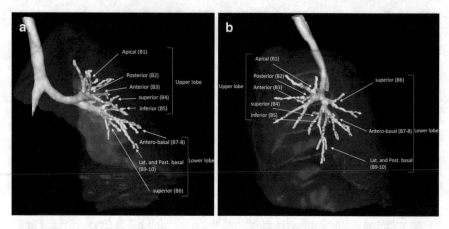

Fig. 1.2 Anatomy of the left bronchus—(**a**) frontal view; (**b**) lateral view (Visible Patient™ software)

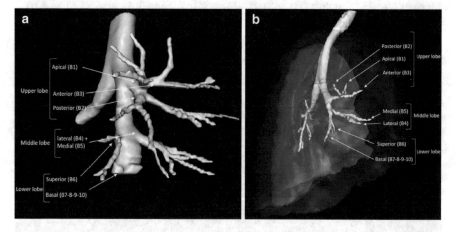

Fig. 1.3 Anatomy of the right bronchus—(**a**) frontal view; (**b**) lateral view (Visible Patient™ software)

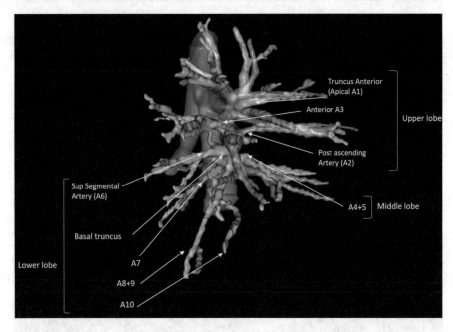

Fig. 1.4 Anatomy of the right pulmonary artery—lateral view (Visible Patient™ software)

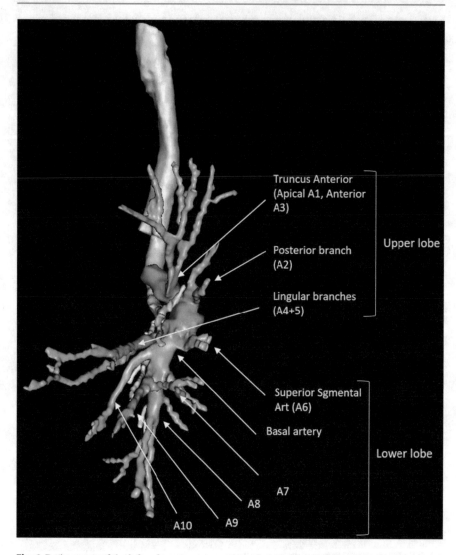

Fig. 1.5 Anatomy of the left pulmonary artery—lateral view (Visible Patient™ software)

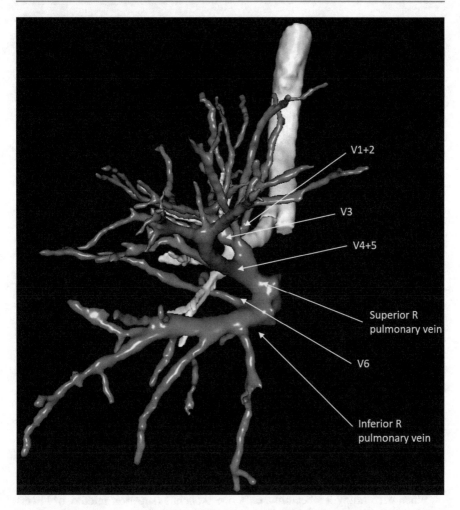

Fig. 1.6 Anatomy of the right pulmonary vein—lateral view (Visible Patient™ software)

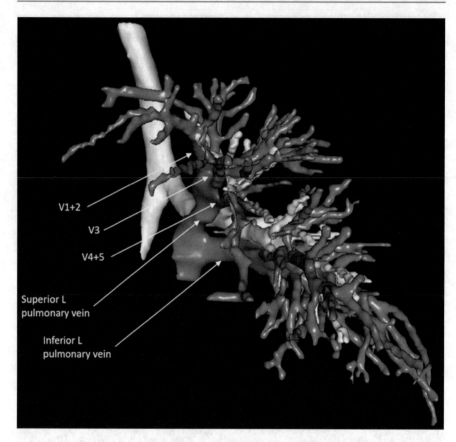

Fig. 1.7 Anatomy of the left pulmonary vein—lateral view (Visible Patient™ software)

When performing a lobectomy, only one bronchus (superior, middle, or lower) and one vein (superior or inferior) usually needs to be controlled. For middle lobectomies, the vein that needs controlling is the inferior branch of the superior pulmonary vein.

Although pulmonary arteries present many variations in location and number, this should not represent a problem when a lobectomy is considered. Indeed, all the arteries coming straight into the lobe should be dissected. Cautiously preserving the vascularization for the remaining lobe is crucial, especially for a proximal lobectomy (upper or middle). In fact, a distal lobectomy (lower) will be technically less challenging than any other lobectomy.

References

1. Morini F, Zani A, Conforti A, et al. Current management of congenital pulmonary airway malformations: a "European Pediatric Surgeons' Association" survey. Eur J Pediatr Surg Off J Austrian Assoc Pediatr Surg Al Z Kinderchir. 2018;28(1):1–5. https://doi.org/10.1055/s-0037-1604020.
2. Aragaki M, Kaga K, Hida Y, Kato T, Matsui Y. Feasibility and safety of reduced-port video-assisted thoracoscopic surgery using a needle scope for pulmonary lobectomy- retrospective study. Ann Med Surg. 2019;45:70–4. https://doi.org/10.1016/j.amsu.2019.07.027.
3. Khosa JK, Leong SL, Borzi PA. Congenital cystic adenomatoid malformation of the lung: indications and timing of surgery. Pediatr Surg Int. 2004;20(7):505–8. https://doi.org/10.1007/s00383-004-1225-4.
4. Naito Y, Beres A, Lapidus-Krol E, Ratjen F, Langer JC. Does earlier lobectomy result in better long-term pulmonary function in children with congenital lung anomalies? A prospective study. J Pediatr Surg. 2012;47(5):852–6. https://doi.org/10.1016/j.jpedsurg.2012.01.037.
5. Clermidi P, Bellon M, Skhiri A, et al. Fast track pediatric thoracic surgery: toward day-case surgery? J Pediatr Surg. 2017;52(11):1800–5. https://doi.org/10.1016/j.jpedsurg.2017.02.005.
6. Boubnova J, Peycelon M, Garbi O, David M, Bonnard A, De Lagausie P. Thoracoscopy in the management of congenital lung diseases in infancy. Surg Endosc. 2011;25(2):593–6. https://doi.org/10.1007/s00464-010-1228-2.
7. Style CC, Mehollin-Ray AR, Verla MA, et al. Accuracy of prenatal and postnatal imaging for management of congenital lung malformations. J Pediatr Surg. 2020;55(5):844–7. https://doi.org/10.1016/j.jpedsurg.2020.01.020.
8. Soler L, Mutter D, Marescaux J. Patient-specific anatomy: the new area of anatomy based on 3D modelling. In: Digital anatomy, Human computer interaction series. Springer; 2021.

References

Technical Considerations and Postoperative Analgesia

2.1 Patient Positioning, Preparation, and Room Setup

Several positions are possible depending on how you decide to approach the vessels in the fissure. The purpose here is not to describe all the different positions, but to describe a position that works for all major resections.

If you decide to approach the fissure perpendicular to the vessels (parallel to the fissure), the child will be placed in lateral decubitus and the operator placed facing the child, with the monitor in the child's back.

If, as performed at our institution, you approach the fissure parallel to the vessels (perpendicular to the fissure), the child will be placed in lateral decubitus, at the end of the table, the operator at the end of the table. The monitor will be placed on the side of the resection, either to the right and top for a right pulmonary resection or to the top and left for a left pulmonary resection (Fig. 2.1).

Supplementary Information The online version contains supplementary material available at [https://doi.org/10.1007/978-3-031-07937-5_2].

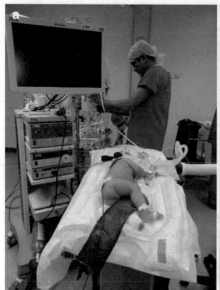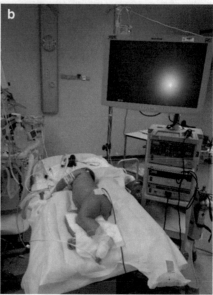

Fig. 2.1 Patient positioning—(**a**) right lobectomy; (**b**) left lobectomy

The advantage of this position is an easier approach for upper lobectomies, allowing access to the upper lobe bronchus on the right; to the vessels and the pulmonary artery by retrograde dissection on the left (see below). The disadvantage of this positioning concerns older children and adolescents for whom this position is not applicable. The position found will therefore be a mix between both positions (see below, section on lobectomies in older children). The 2 positions are in my opinion equivalent as long as they are acquired and practiced frequently by the operator.

In both cases, it will be necessary to clear the shoulder well and place the homolateral arm upwards to tilt the scapula forward, which is an important landmark for the insertion of the first trocar.

The positioning of the child on the operating table will be done in close collaboration with the anesthesia team and after all the prothesis (intravenous access and endotracheal tube) have been correctly inserted. In the vast majority of cases, selective intubation is not necessary. Indeed, since the surgery is aimed for children under 5 months of age, selective intubation would have to be obtained using a bronchial blocker, whose placement may be challenging for a team not familiar with this technique. In adolescents, selective ventilation may be more easily obtained using selective intubation tubes.

In order to bypass the need for selective ventilation, CO_2 insufflation will be necessary in order to collapse the lung and obtain a satisfactory workspace. At our institution, an insufflation pressure of 5 mmHg is used, but some teams choose pressures as high as 8 or 10 mmHg without encountering any difficulties. The flow rate will not exceed 1.5 ml/min. It should be kept in mind that there is on the one hand a mediastinal deviation induced by insufflation and on the other hand a resorption of CO_2 which will therefore induce hypercapnia (metabolic acidosis). This can be compensated using ventilation, by increasing ventilation frequencies in order to increase the clearance of CO_2. The ideal, however, is to ensure that the ventilation volumes are not too important in order to maintain an adequate working space. Any positive expiratory pressure (PEP) is always suppressed, in order to allow the lung, compressed by the insufflation of CO_2, to be collapsed and thus gain working space. This technique, without the use of bronchial blockers or selective intubation, also allows to ventilate the child quickly either in the event of desaturation or on demand, for example, to perform a leak test after controlling a bronchus or after a parenchymal section. At the start of insufflation, mild desaturation and temporary hypercapnia are frequent, and will gradually be corrected once the adaptative mechanisms, such as an increase in cardiac output, are established. This often allows the child to be correctly ventilated. The anesthesiologist usually tolerates a permissive hypercapnia about 55 mmHg allowing sufficient working space to perform the procedure. The placement of a NIRS sensor (Near Infrared Spectroscopy) on the forehead allows an optimization of the intraoperative monitoring in these children [1, 2].

Even if the thorax provides an incompressible workspace due to the rigidity of the rib cage, it is also preferable to paralyze the child. Indeed, this avoids intrathoracic incursion of the diaphragm which can interfere with dissection, especially of the inferior pulmonary vein.

A gastric tube will be systematically inserted. Indeed, for reasons that are not fully explained, postoperative gastric distension is frequent after thoracoscopic pulmonary resections. It can be removed immediately at the end of the surgery, after complete gastric emptying, especially if the child is in an enhanced recovery circuit.

Finally, the necessity to convert to thoracotomy should always be considered. The drapes should therefore be placed accordingly, that is to say on the spine line behind and clearing the nipple at the front. At the bottom, enough room should be left for drainage.

2.2 Instrumentation

As already mentioned above, all the instruments must be checked with the operating room nurse before beginning the procedure.

2.2.1 Thoracoscopy Instruments

Instruments of either 3 or 5 mm can be used. Three or 4 trocars will be needed. Given the small workspace, 30° optical lens seems more suitable than 0°. It allows you to have a view "from above" rather than low-angled. Most often, two nontraumatic grasping forceps (Fig. 2.2), or a Maryland type forceps, a dissector, and a needle holder (Fig. 2.3) will be sufficient. Our preference goes to 5-mm instruments in this surgery for several reasons.

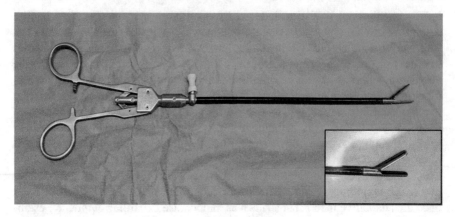

Fig. 2.2 Grasper forceps (Storz endoscopie, Guyancourt, France)

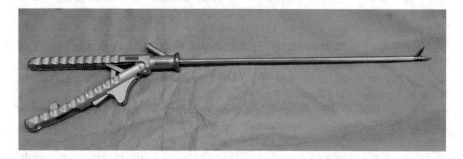

Fig. 2.3 Needle holder (Ethicon Endosurgery, Issy-Les-Moulineaux, France)

The first trocar introduced is initially used for the 5-mm optical in order to introduce the other trocars under direct visual control, but the optical will then be placed in another location for the surgery, which makes another 5-mm trocar necessary.

Whereas thermofusion instruments are available in 3 and 5 mm, we prefer using the 5-mm, as the 3-mm does not allow sectioning, which complicates and lengthens the surgery in the event of a necessary parenchymal section.

Additionally, you must be able to use both your left hand and your right hand alternatively, and therefore be able to exchange the instruments you use in both hands, requiring identical port size in both operating ports.

Finally, if you want to use the 5-mm mechanical stapler you will need a 5-mm port.

For all these reasons we prefer to use 5-mm instruments.

Of course, Thoracoport™ (Covidien, Dublin, Ireland) should not be used in this technique, as it is necessary to insufflate and therefore use tap trocars.

Trocars should be secured in order to prevent the trocars from being mobilized out of the thorax unexpectedly but also too far inside the thoracic cavity, which would obstruct the opening of the instruments. A Mersuture™ type thread (Ethicon, Cincinnati, USA) or silk thread (Ethicon, Cincinnati, USA) is used to fix the trocar to the wall and prevent its mobilization out of the thorax.

Several methods are possible in order to prevent the trocar to be mobilized inside the thoracic cavity: a previously sterilized Rilsan, a latex catheter threaded on the trocar (i.e., red rubber catheter), or a steristrip (Fig. 2.4).

Fig. 2.4 Trocar is secured to avoid dislodgment

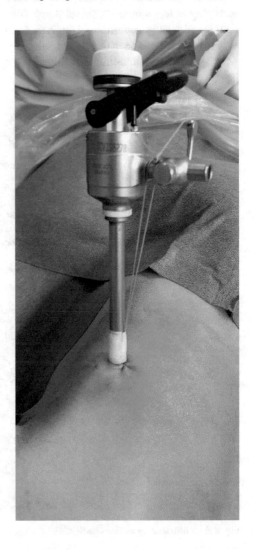

2.2.2 Hemostasis Instruments

The monopolar hook or the bipolar forceps are hardly used any more since the development of thermofusion forceps (Ligasure™, Covidien, Minneapolis, USA or Enseal®, Ethicon, Cincinnati, USA) (Fig. 2.5). Some models (Maryland type) allow both the dissection of the vessels to be carried out in complete safety, as well as the parenchymal section, and efficient aerostasis. Ultracision (Harmonic Synergy®, Ethicon, Cincinnati, USA) can also be used for the parenchymal section, but its extremity is less suited for vessel dissection and has an extremely hot jaw that can damage adjacent structures and the vessels themselves. Recently, a 3-mm thermofusion instrument has been developed, allowing the operation to be carried out entirely with 3-mm instrumentation (JustRight™ Surgical, Boulder, USA) (Fig. 2.6).

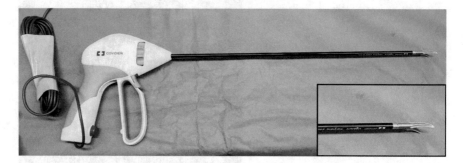

Fig. 2.5 Ligasure™ (Covidien, Minneapolis, USA)

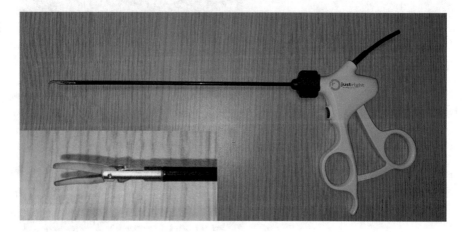

Fig. 2.6 3-mm sealing device (JustRight™ Surgical, Boulder, USA)

Finally, an absorbable suture (Vicryl™, Ethicon, Cincinnati, USA) of 2/0 and 3/0 will be necessary for ligatures. A suture thread of PDS® or Vicryl™ 4/0 or 5/0 (Ethicon, Cincinnati, USA) with needle may also be necessary to complete hemostasis or aerostasis.

2.2.3 Mechanical Stapler

The most commonly commercialized mechanical staples, i.e., 10 mm, should not be used, as a 12-mm trocar would be required, which is not reasonable in an infant of 3 to 5 months of age. The 5-mm stapler (Justright™ surgical, Boulder, USA) (Fig. 2.7) can be used to control the vein and bronchus, or even a slightly bulky basal trunk, or to complete an incomplete fissure. It safely and efficiently performs aerostasis, as long as the instructions are strictly followed in order to avoid incomplete stapling [3].

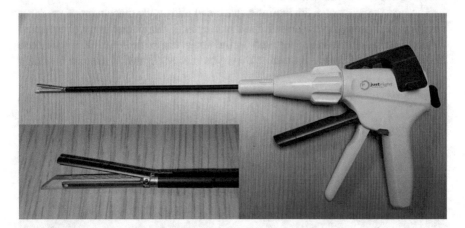

Fig. 2.7 5-mm mechanical stapler (JustRight™ Surgical, Boulder, USA)

2.2.4 Endobag

The use of an Endobag is not essential but removing the resected pulmonary tissue through a 3- or 5-mm incision will necessarily require splitting it. The risk is therefore to leave fragments in the thorax which can be a factor of postoperative adhesions. In order to avoid this, a 5-mm or 10-mm Endobag can be used, ideally placed in the most posterior incision, which is the less visible incision.

2.3   Placement and Positioning of the Trocars

The positioning of the trocars in this technique should in no way replace the positioning already acquired by those who perform major pulmonary resections under thoracoscopy. The positioning of the trocars ensues from the positioning of the child and obeys the fundamentals of laparoscopy: work in the axis of the structure you want to dissect and triangulation.

The first trocar creates the working space and allows the placement of the other trocars under visual control (Fig. 2.8). It is inserted 1 cm under the tip of the scapula, in the fifth intercostal space, and on the upper edge of the rib. Once you have made sure you are in the thoracic cavity, you can begin insufflation at 5 mmHg

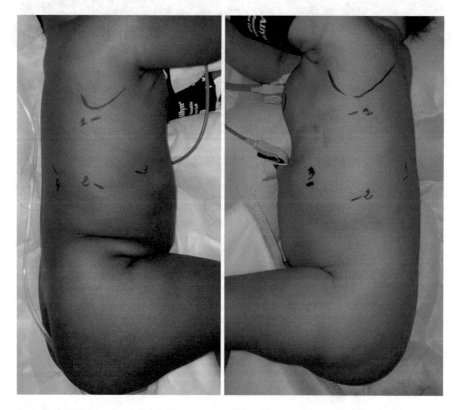

Fig. 2.8 Placement of the trocars. The numbers represent the placement order

which will allow the lung to collapse. In this first trocar, the 30° optical is inserted. It is then necessary to visualize the diaphragm, using the 30° angulation by turning the optical upside down. A second trocar is then inserted on the same line as the first, immediately above the insertion of the diaphragm. The optical is then placed in this latest trocar for the rest of the surgery. Two other trocars will be inserted on either side of this one, respecting a good triangulation, always immediately above the insertion of the diaphragm. The anterior trocar should be placed approximately on the anterior axillary line and the posterior trocar on the posteriori axillary line without going too close to the spine because the ribs get closer and may limit the mobility of the instrument.

The trocars will be secured as previously described. The first trocar will be used to recline structures or exposition if necessary (Movie 2.1).

2.4   Vascular Control: Bleeding Management

In most of the lobectomy techniques that will be described, vascular, arterial, or venous control is often the first step. Only the upper right lobectomy will be an exception. Moreover, arterial control often precedes venous control.

Dissection of the artery follows the same rules as in open surgery. Dissection should be performed in the lining of the artery, as close as possible to the artery, in order to ensure the efficiency of the thermofusion systems. Whereas some surgeons use only thermofusion (Ligasure, Enseal) to control the artery, others prefer using a 5-mm mechanical stapler, especially large basal trunks. A safe technique is proximal ligation with an absorbable suture (Vicryl 2/0 or 3/0), followed by a gentle traction on the knot that allows the dissection to be carried downstream, towards the bifurcation branches. These latter branches being of a smaller caliber, control and section will be safely performed using thermofusion (Movie 2.2).

In parallel, the systemic arteries of a sequestration would be controlled the same way. The dissection of the artery should be carried out as closely as possible to the artery, which will be ligatured using Vicryl 2/0 or 3/0, followed by section and/or thermofusion as far as possible in the parenchyma. An Endoloop can be placed for additional safety (Movie 2.3).

Venous control follows the same rules of dissection. As this is a low-pressure system, Ligasure is usually sufficient on its own. The dissection is carried out as proximally as possible, in order to control the smaller branches. A safe technique is to fuse on both sides and then cut between both fusion areas, initially partially in order to ensure the absence of bleeding. If there is any bleeding, thermofusion may be performed on both areas before completing the section. Using the current Ligasure forceps can allow us to overcome this maneuver. The dissection should be carried sufficiently in order to leave a long enough stump before its penetration into the pericardium. This security enables us to complete the hemostasis, either with ligasure™ or by means of a ligation, if a bleeding occurs once the vein has been sectioned (Movies 2.4 and 2.5).

In the event of arterial bleeding, two errors must be avoided absolutely:

- Aspiration as this will immediately reventilate the lung which will completely hide the origin of the bleeding.
- Asking your assistant to come closer with the camera with a risk of projection on the camera and therefore total loss of vision.

The old adage "prevention is better than cure" applies perfectly here. Indeed, if the dissection has been carried out with special care and the vessels are well individualized, the occurrence of bleeding should not be a problem and is in no way a reason for conversion to open surgery. Bleeding can be controlled either using Ligasure provided that it is at a distance from the original vessel that we want to respect (and therefore that the dissection has been perfect) or by means of a Vicryl 4/0, 5/0 or PDS 5/0 knot (Movie 2.6).

If bleeding occurs during the dissection, the urgent maneuver is to stop the bleeding with the grasper used for the dissection. Once this is done, you need to think about what would be the next step: try to do the hemostasis with a vessel sealer device or use a stitch. Most often, the dissection needs to be completed and pushed forward with the other hand while the grasper is stopping the bleeding. It is the only way to correctly visualize the origin of the bleeding. It is also a way to move away from the vessel we want to respect doing the hemostasis. Once the origin of the bleeding has been identified, it is easy to use an absorbable suture or a sealing device (Movie 2.7).

If venous bleeding occurs, the issue is different depending on if the bleeding is originating from the parenchyma, from a small intralobar branch, or even from a small branch upstream of an inferior or superior pulmonary vein or from the pulmonary vein itself.

In the first case, the Ligasure will most often control the bleeding.

In the second case, if the bleeding is related to an injury of the upper or lower pulmonary vein, the CO_2 insufflation should be first stopped in order to avoid CO_2 embolism, followed by clamping of the vein or the wound in order to stop the bleeding. Once the bleeding has been controlled, the best thing in my opinion is not to use the Ligasure. Indeed, if the thermofusion is incomplete and the vein disappears in the pericardium, controlling the bleeding will become difficult. Instead, a stitch of vicryl 4/0 or 5/0 should be used to close the tear (Movie 2.8).

2.5   Bronchial Control: Management of Air Leaks

The safest way for bronchial control is obviously mechanical stapling, using a 5-mm mechanical stapler. However, the control of this bronchus obeys the same rules of dissection as vascular structures. Even if the control of the bronchus appears easier before the vein, both structures are intimately linked and it is therefore necessary to separate the vein behind the bronchus in order to avoid a joint control, which could result in a vasculo-bronchial fistula. For this reason, the vein should be controlled first, followed by bronchial control.

Even once the bronchus is completely dissected, care should be taken in order to avoid ligation of the main bronchus. For this, the key is to dissect downstream extensively, until the different bifurcation branches. At this point, the difficulty is to control the different branches, without leaving open a small bifurcation branch that could be unnoticed and whose leakage may be difficult to control or even identify. If in doubt, a clamping test may be performed, by asking the anesthesiologist to reventilate the lung. In addition, during the dissection of the bronchus using mono- or bipolar coagulation, some tissue should be left around, in order to avoid devascularization that may result in broncho-pleural fistula.

Ligation of the bronchus in children is safely done using an absorbable suture such as vicryl 2/0 or 3/0. The bronchus is then sectioned without distal ligating. A shot of prophylactic antibiotics may be administered at this time of the procedure. Care will be taken to reventilate the lung and perform a leak test after section (Movies 2.9 and 2.10).

An easier and faster control may be performed using a mechanical stapler. However, an incomplete closure of the bronchus may occur if the stapler is not used properly.

If an air leak occurs, it should first be identified. It may be challenging to differentiate a parenchymal air leak coming from the separation of the lobes (complete fissure) from a leak originating from a branch of division, which can be very small in a 3–4-month-old baby.

Postoperatively, both types of leaks may be differentiated by the type of bubbling.

For a parenchymal leak, the bubbling will be intermittent, and the leak will tend to spontaneously heal. Patience will be required.

In the leak originates from a division branch, the bubbling will be constant and continuous, starting in the recovery room. The whole line and connection of the drain should be first checked in order to ensure the absence of leak at this level. A systematic chest X-ray will then be performed in the recovery room and will often show a pneumothorax. In this case, it is best to take the child back to the OR before leaving the recovery room in order to complete the aerostasis.

After identifying the leak, a stitch of vicryl 4/0 or 5/0 (or PDS) will be placed, until a completely satisfactory leak test is obtained (Movie 2.11).

2.6 Drainage

The question of drainage is currently a matter of debate, in particular for issues of analgesia and outpatient care. The size of drains used for 3–4 months old children will not exceed 10 or 12 CH. For pulmonary malformation resection, the reduction in the number of drains from 2 to 1 is now commonly accepted. This is probably not the case all the time when it comes to performing a lobar resection for bronchiectasis or for an infectious process, such as a fungal infection in an immunocompromised patient for example.

Nowadays, the question of drainage itself is still questionable. Indeed, for extralobar sequestrations, a drain is no longer used at our institution. For intralobar sequestrations, a drain will not be used if an atypical resection has been performed, as long as the aerostasis is satisfactory. For major lobar resections, if the bronchus has been correctly controlled and the hemostasis is satisfactory as described above with a complete fissure, drainage is not essential. The exception remains for lobectomies performed for giant lobar emphysema. When removed late, these voluminous lobes may have chronically compressed the adjacent lobes, inducing pulmonary hypoplasia and a significant mediastinal shift. For these reasons, these children may behave as neonates with congenital diaphragmatic hernia (CDH). Drainage will help re-expand the remaining lobes and reduce the mediastinal shift. Sudden refocusing of the mediastinum should be avoided as in CDH, and the vacant space may become filled by pleural effusion that must be respected.

Regarding drainage, gentle suction is applied during the first 24 hours, between -10 and -15 cm H_2O. The day after the surgery, in the absence of bubbling, suction is discontinued, and the drain is left on water seal. The drain is then removed a few hours later if the child is well. A chest X-ray will only be performed once the drain has been removed. Indeed, the X-ray before drain removal shows postoperative changes that should not be a reason to continue the drainage (see below).

As a conclusion, either no drain is used or, if a drain is used, it should be removed the morning after the surgery, with the only exception being emphysema.

Postoperative pneumothorax may be observed in undrained children while the aerostasis controlled during the operation was perfect. Almost all of these children present with subcutaneous emphysema postoperatively which resolves rapidly within 24–48 h. It is possible that the resorption of this emphysema inside the pleural cavity causes this pneumothorax. Most often, a 24-h drainage will solve the problem.

References

1. Yu LS, Lei YQ, Liu JF, et al. A comparison between selective lobar bronchial blockade and main bronchial blockade in pediatric thoracoscopic surgery: a retrospective cohort study. J Cardiothorac Vasc Anesth. 2022;36(2):518–23. https://doi.org/10.1053/j.jvca.2021.09.002.
2. Huang J, Cao H, Chen Q, et al. The comparison between bronchial occlusion and artificial pneumothorax for thoracoscopic lobectomy in infants. J Cardiothorac Vasc Anesth. 2021;35(8):2326–9. https://doi.org/10.1053/j.jvca.2020.11.014.
3. Rothenberg S. Thoracoscopic lobectomy in infants and children utilizing a 5 mm stapling device. J Laparoendosc Adv Surg Tech A. 2016;26(12):1036–8. https://doi.org/10.1089/lap.2016.0334.

"Tips and Tricks" and Management of Peroperative Difficulties and Complications

3.1   I Need to Ventilate because the Child Is Desaturating

This is usually the first problem that occurs at the beginning of the procedure. Indeed, insufflation with CO_2 compresses the lung and can interfere with the superior vena cava return. The contralateral lung is also hampered by the support placed under the child. There is therefore often a desaturation from the insufflation. Communication with the anesthesiologist is crucial. If the anesthesiologist increases ventilation pressures or volumes, the workspace will significantly decrease and it will become more difficult to work. Desaturation is often transient, until the adaptation mechanisms, such as an increase in the heart rate, are triggered. The child may be ventilated with 100% FiO_2 if necessary. Likewise, hypercapnia is often present. It will also be necessary to know how to tolerate a permissive hypercapnia around 50–60 mmHg. If necessary, the anesthesiologist and the surgeon will have to find a compromise with ventilatory parameters which allows oxygenation, satisfactory CO_2 clearance, and a sufficient workspace. In this situation, the fourth trocar is particularly useful by correctly exposing the part of the lung to be dissected by pushing the adjacent lung away if necessary.

Supplementary Information The online version contains supplementary material available at [https://doi.org/10.1007/978-3-031-07937-5_3].

Selective intubation is used by some teams, but it may result in atelectasis and postoperative ventilation issues. A Fogarty catheter may be used to inflate the balloon in the main bronchus. This may be difficult to place and often results in migration of the balloon. Although our experience does not report these benefits, bronchial occlusion has been reported to offer an improved surgical exposure, a shorter operative time, decreased intraoperative bleeding, and a shorter duration of tracheal intubation [1]. Selective blockers have also been used to avoid postoperative atelectasis. We do not have any experience with selective blockers at our institution.

3.2   I Have No Space to Work

This issue often arises from the initial problems of desaturation. As explained above, this should be transient. If there is no improvement, several things need to be checked:

- Ask the anesthesiologist if the PEP (positive expiratory pressure) has been removed, as PEP would prevent lung decompression and therefore take up workspace.
- If the anesthesiologist needs to maintain high insufflation pressures, it is necessary to verify that the child is not selectively intubated on the side of the lobectomy. This would result in the absence of ventilation of the contralateral lung, explaining the desaturation and need for high pressures. Removing the endotracheal tube a few centimeters would then be necessary.
- If despite this the workspace issue persists, the child may need to be aspirated. Indeed, a mucous plug may compromise ventilation on the contralateral lung.
- Ensure that the child is fully paralyzed in order to limit the movements of the diaphragm which can interfere with the surgery.
- Decompress large cysts that can interfere with the dissection by piercing them.
- If you are using a selective ventilation, the lung should be decompressed using artificial pneumothorax and CO_2 insufflation before inflating the blocker in the bronchus. If the bronchial blocker is inflated first, it will be impossible to decompress the lung afterwards.

3.3   My Fissure Is Complete

Before beginning the dissection, the surgeon should first check whether the fissure is complete or not. In order to complete a fissure, you have to find the arterial plane. Once it is found, all structures that are in front of this plane may be sectioned without any risk. This may include some interlobar veins that can be coagulated without any consequence. On both sides, completing the posterior side of the fissure involves the risk of injuring the superior segmental artery. It is therefore safer to start the posterior dissection of the fissure from the lateral edge of this artery.

Completing the anterior side of the fissure is usually safe, provided that the superior and inferior pulmonary veins are identified and respected. On the right, this maneuver usually allows you to quickly reach the medial edge of the basal trunk and then open the visceral pleura in front of it. On the left, it will enable to reach either the anterior lingular artery or the basal trunk.

The minor fissure is more difficult to complete and the plane between the middle lobe and the upper lobe may be challenging to identify. For this reason, completing the minor fissure is usually the last step to perform, both for upper and middle lobectomies. Indeed, the prior control of the bronchus of the concerned lobe allows clear identification of the fissure and facilitates its dissection starting from the arterial plane.

3.4   It Is Bleeding and I Cannot See

This is what makes this surgery possibly scary for some surgeons. Pulmonary arteries may bleed massively and compromise the operative field, quickly making the situation out of control. A thoracotomy set, a Finochietto retractor, and vascular clamps should always be available in the operating room.

Some simple rules can apply to avoid these situations:

- Have a good understanding of the lung anatomy and its vascularization.
- Perform a perfect dissection of the arteries, and avoid "en masse" coagulation or stapling without dissection. This will allow to easily control the bleeding by clamping the artery with forceps.
- If there is bleeding, avoid prolonged aspiration: this would result in loss of workspace and vision due to pulmonary inflation, but may quickly lead to hypovolemia in a baby with a blood mass of 80 ml/kg and only about 500 ml for a 6-kg baby. Tamponade, either by forceps or if necessary, with a piece of dressing that you have passed through a port, should be preferred.
- Once the bleeding has stopped and its origin has been identified, controlling it using a clip or a knot should be straightforward, as long as the artery has been dissected properly. If this is not the case, the bleeding may be controlled using one hand, while the other may push the dissection a little further to create space for a clip or knot. Always remember that this kind of situation is at high risk of resulting in iatrogenic complications by injuring structures, such as the phrenic nerve and bronchus. In order to avoid this situation, the dissection should be pursued sufficiently in order to be able to control any bleeding. If, despite all this, you are unable to achieve hemostasis, conversion will be necessary. Before performing the thoracotomy, the bleeding should always be controlled with grasping forceps.
- The pulmonary veins will be dissected and controlled so as to leave a sufficiently large stump outside the pericardium. If there is bleeding on the stump, this length will be useful for control.

3.5   I Cannot Find My Artery

Sometimes, often due to complete fissures, it is difficult to find the arteries and especially the main artery deeply in the fissure. When trying to find it, you will sometimes manage to find what undoubtedly corresponds to a branch of this artery: a lingular branch, a segmental branch, etc. It can then be useful to place a stay stitch around this artery, in order to gently put it in tension with one hand, and continue the dissection proximally with the other hand until you find your main artery at the level of the fissure (Movie 3.1).

3.6   I Don't Recognize the Anatomy

This should not happen if you took the time to prepare your procedure. With the help of the tips given above, you should be able to find at least one artery, follow it and locate the main artery deep in the fissure. Never cut anything without knowing exactly what it is!

3.7   I Cannot Find My Minor Fissure

This can happen for a right upper lobectomy or a middle lobectomy. This is where controlling the bronchus before trying to separate the upper lobe from the middle lobe is crucial. If each step is respected, the bronchus would have been already controlled before arriving at the stage of the fissure. You can then ask the anesthesiologist to ventilate the child and you can stop insufflating the CO_2. You should see the dividing line corresponding to the fissure between the ventilated lobe and the unventilated lobe (either the middle lobe or the upper lobe). It is necessary to start the dissection of the fissure starting from the artery at the intersection between the large fissure and the small fissure.

3.8   My Remaining Lobe Is Not Ventilating Well

This is probably the worst thing that can happen after a lobectomy. Several things have to be checked:

- The insufflation of CO_2 should be stopped and the pneumothorax aspirated to help with lung expansion.
- The absence of leakage originating from a bronchial stump.
- The child has been aspirated to remove a mucous plug that could block the bronchus.

- Positive expiratory pressure has been applied again.
- You have checked the anatomy at the level of the hilum, in particular the bronchial stump in order to eliminate any problem at the level of the remaining bronchi.

If despite this the lung does not reventilate, it is necessary to push the exploration and ask for a peroperative bronchial endoscopy to rule out any issue with the bronchi.

It is very rare that no cause is found. The only possible cause after eliminating any problem is a distal obliterating disease that results in obliteration of the distal endings of the bronchial division. This is often post-viral and can result in a lobar bronchiectasis that may require a lobectomy.

Reference

1. Huang J, Cao H, Chen Q, et al. The comparison between bronchial occlusion and artificial pneumothorax for thoracoscopic lobectomy in infants. J Cardiothorac Vasc Anesth. 2021;35(8):2326–9. https://doi.org/10.1053/j.jvca.2020.11.014.

Further Reading

Gossot D. Atlas of endoscopic major pulmonary resections. Springer; 2018. libgen.lc.

Postoperative Management: Chest-X-Ray—Management of Complications and Postoperative Pain—Follow-Up

4

4.1 Postoperative Chest X-Ray

Pulmonary malformation resection may be complicated by ventilatory issues, pneumothorax, or pleural effusion. At our institution, we carried out a study on a series of patients operated on for congenital pulmonary malformation by thoracoscopy until 2012 (unpublished data). The aim of this study was to report early postoperative radiological changes and their evolution. Chest X-rays performed on postoperative day (POD) 2 and POD30 were retrospectively reviewed. Only patients operated on between 2007 and 2012 for congenital lobar emphysema (CLE), adenomatoid malformation (CCAM), or intralobar sequestration (ILS) were included. Postoperative radiological changes were classified in four grades of increasing severity (0, 1, 2, and 3). Overall, 55 patients underwent thoracoscopic surgery, and 35 were included (26 CCAM, 8 CLE, and 1 ILS). On POD2, 6 patients presented stage 0 and 1 lesions, 26 patients with stage 2 and 3 lesions. On POD30, 24 patients had stable (68.6%) stage 2 lesions, 10 improved to a stage of severity lower (28.6%) and 1 worsened (2.8%). The median hospital stay was similar for stages 0–1, and 2 (3.4 and 3 days respectively). Only patients classified as stage 3 on POD2 had an increased median hospital stay (8 days).

The chest X-ray after pulmonary resection was rarely normal on POD2. In two thirds of the cases it did not improve by D30. However, the median hospital stay was the same for patients classified as stage 0, 1, or 2 and therefore was not a reason for longer hospitalization. For this reason, patients in our center have two chest X-rays: one at the end of the procedure in the recovery room, and another the day after the surgery, before the drain removal and discharge. Patients who are operated on as a day case surgery without a drain would have only one chest X-ray in the recovery room.

In conclusion, surgeon should not decide on the length of hospital stay based on the chest X-ray findings.

We have seen the most frequent intraoperative complications and their management. Postoperative complications can be divided into the categories.

4.2 Immediate Complications (Recovery Room)

These complications occur early, starting in the recovery room. Patients who have undergone pulmonary resections should always be seen by the surgeon being discharged to the ward.

4.2.1 Bubbling in the Chest Tube

As mentioned above, the first reflex when confronted with bubbling should be to check the whole drainage line for any technical issues and leakage. Once this is ruled out, the continuous or intermittent nature of the bubbling will help you decide on the need for immediate reintervention.

4.2.2 Bleeding or Oozing of Postoperative Secretions Through the Openings of the Trocars

Although this is a frequent event that can get you called to the recovery room, it is rarely pure blood, but most often postoperative secretions, and sometimes some effusion remaining from lavage. A compressive dressing is often sufficient.

4.2.3 Subcutaneous Emphysema (Clinical and Radiological)

Subcutaneous emphysema is present in almost all cases of thoracoscopic pulmonary resections. Its extensive nature should raise suspicion of a bronchial leak, especially when no drainage is present. The presence of subcutaneous emphysema should be closely monitored, but it is most often nonevolutive and spontaneously resolves.

4.2.4 Accidental Removal of the Nasogastric Tube

Every child that undergoes a thoracoscopy presents with a postoperative gastric distension, whose origin is not completely elucidated. The patient usually arrives in the recovery room with a gastric tube, whose accidental removal is a frequent reason for being called to the recovery room. There is no need to place another gastric tube.

To avoid this incident, the nasogastric tube can be removed in the operating room, as soon as the procedure is finished, after having completely aspirated and emptied the stomach.

4.2.5 Postoperative Pneumothorax (PNO)

This is the only pathological finding on the postoperative X-ray that deserves attention. As mentioned above, postoperative images related to a hematoma of the pulmonary parenchyma or ventilation disorders are frequent, but do not constitute complications as themselves. Postoperative pneumothorax is common after surgery for emphysema. It will be necessary to verify that suction is active on the drainage, and that there is no bubbling. If the drain is bubbling, a surgical reintervention should be considered. If there is no bubbling, expectative management can be preferred. In this case, the pneumothorax should be monitored using serial X-rays.

4.3 Complications During the Hospital Stay

4.3.1 Persistent Bubbling

This is the most common complication. If the drain still bubbles after a few days, suction should be stopped and the drain should be left on water seal, in case there is a parenchymal leak in contact with the drain itself. A chest X-ray should be performed after stopping suction in order to verify the absence of pneumothorax occurrence. Often, if the bubbling stops, the drain will be gradually mobilized before being completely removed. If a pneumothorax appears after stopping the suction, suction should be applied again for a few more days. It is rare that a parenchymal leak does not heal spontaneously.

4.3.2 Persistent Pneumothorax Despite Drainage

This is the prerogative of giant lobar emphysema, operated late, with "chronic" mediastinal deviation, a mass effect on the adjacent lobes with a certain degree of hypoplasia. The remaining lung has difficulty returning to the wall despite the drain. A second drain is often placed, but often with little effect. Sometimes an effusion will fill the pleural cavity, as in children with CDH. You have to know how to be patient. Patients may be discharged without a drain, but with a minor pneumothorax.

Sometimes the drain is clogged. We do not like the classic drain "milking" maneuver that offers extremely large negative depression that can damage the lung or any other structure in contact with the drain. We have had satisfying results with the use of Actilyse according to the following protocol (based on studies of the use of Actilyse in infectious pleuro-pneumonia):

Actilyse Protocol
Minimal weight = 5 kg
   Minimal age = 3 months
   Dosage = 0.1 mg/kg with a max of 3 mg diluted in a volume of 10 to 30 ml of saline
   Most frequent dosage = 2 mg (Maximum dosage = 4 to 5 mg)
   Dilution volume = 10 to 100 ml (0.1 mg/ml)
   Clamping time = 45 min to 4 h
   Number of doses = Repeated/8 h or 12 h or x1/day
   Duration of treatment = 3 to 4 days (up to 10 doses) or maximum of 3–6 doses
   Criteria to stop = drainage volume < 25 ml/12 h or < 40 ml/24 h

The use of Actilyse may help unclog the drain and reexpand the lung back to the wall. It should be noted that there is no published literature on the use of Actilyse in the potential presence of a broncho-pleural fistula.

Finally, it happens that the lung does not return to the wall, with a constant bubbling. In this case, it is indeed necessary to think about a broncho-pleural fistula. If the diagnosis has not been made in the recovery room but is delayed several days after surgery, we will have to consider a surgical reintervention. A pleuro-empyema is frequent and makes challenging both the dissection and the identification of the location of the leak. An intraoperative bronchial endoscopy can be useful, on the one hand, to identify the leak visually or by opacification, and on the other hand, to catheterize the fistula using a guide wire exteriorized in the pleural cavity. This latter procedure will help identify the fistula during the surgical reintervention. Expectative management can also be an option. Do not expect to have a normal x-ray in this case. Actually, pneumothorax can still be present while the patient is doing well and despite the drain you placed. In this case, the patient can be discharged and followed in outpatient clinic. It will take many months to the chest X-ray to normalize (around 6 months, or more, in our experience).

4.3.3   Bloody Drainage

This should not happen if vascular control is rigorously verified at the end of the procedure, especially in the presence of a sequestration systemic artery. Remember: a knot is always better than a clip or the use of sealing device "en masse" without a good dissection of the vascular structure. If this occurs, obviously you will need to check the hemodynamic status (heart rate, mean arterial pressure, urine output), the hemoglobin, and the drain output every hour. If the patient is unstable, requiring a fluid challenge or transfusion, the indication for surgical reintervention is formal. The surgical approach depends on the stability of the patient, and on the surgeon's confidence with either thoracoscopy or thoracotomy. Most often, the surgeon's preference will go towards a thoracotomy, but a thoracoscopic approach can be safely used, especially if the bleeding is not "cataclysmic."

4.4 Pain Management

Pain management is started in the operating room. The systematic use of a paravertebral analgesia catheter placed at the end of the thoracoscopy by the surgeon has radically changed pain management of patients undergoing thoracic surgery. A paravertebral catheter is inserted percutaneously under thoracoscopic vision at the end of the surgical procedure (Tuohy epidural kit, Perifix ONE Paed set 20®). The thoracoscopic control allows to visualize the tip of the needle in the paravertebral space, without breaching the parietal pleura. An indwelling catheter is then placed under direct vision and can be used to inject local anesthetics (Levobupivacaine 0.25 mL/Kg) with intravenous adjuncts drugs (clonidine or dexamethasone). The catheter can then be removed in day case surgeries or left in place with a continuous infusion if the patient is hospitalized with a drain. These drug adjuncts were used in purpose of improving the quality and duration of the block, according to a multimodal analgesia protocol [1–4].

Once the catheter is removed, pain management is switched to oral medication, such as paracetamol and NSAIDs, in order to allow discharge. A last bolus is performed before removal of the catheter on POD1 before discharge.

Using this protocol, postoperative pain is well controlled, avoiding ventilation issues and postoperative atelectasis. Patients can start feeding a few hours after surgery.

4.5 Follow-Up

Postoperative follow-up should be standardized as much as possible in order to homogenize the series for analysis and interpretation of the outcome. At our institution, a multidisciplinary outpatient clinic, including a pediatric pulmonologist, gastroenterologist, psychomotor therapist, and surgeon, was initially created for esophageal atresia (EA) patients, in the context of the EA national plan. We decided to integrate patients with CPAM to these multidisciplinary clinics, in order to standardize the pulmonary follow-up.

Postoperative	1 month	3 months	6 months	1 year	2 years	3 years	6 years	Every 2 years
Surgeon	X	X			X	X		X
Multidisciplinary team			X	X			X	X
Chest X-ray	X							
Pulmonary function test							X	

Outpatient clinic at 1 month and 3 months is carried out by the surgeon alone (apart from cases that have been complicated during hospitalization). An X-ray is usually performed systematically 1 month after surgery. If this is normal or subnormal, there is no need for further radiological controls. If necessary, a chest X-ray can be repeated at 3 months.

During these two consultations, pulmonary issues must be detected. Indeed, some patients will develop bronchial hyperresponsiveness or pulmonary infections, most often viral (11% in our series, unpublished results). The high rate of bronchial hyperresponsiveness suggests a defect in bronchial organogenesis of the whole lung beside the malformation. In the occurrence of bronchial hyperresponsiveness, the patient will be seen as early as 6 months after surgery in a multidisciplinary outpatient clinic. Otherwise, the multidisciplinary clinic will be planned at 1 year after surgery. The follow-up will then be adapted according to the clinical condition of the child. A systematic pulmonary function test will be performed at the age of 6.

References

1. Karmakar MK. Thoracic paravertebral block. Anesthesiology. 2001;95(3):771–80. https://doi.org/10.1097/00000542-200109000-00033.
2. Karmakar MK, Gin T, Ho AM. Ipsilateral thoraco-lumbar anaesthesia and paravertebral spread after low thoracic paravertebral injection. Br J Anaesth. 2001;87(2):312–6. https://doi.org/10.1093/bja/87.2.312.
3. Kaiser AM, Zollinger A, De Lorenzi D, Largiadèr F, Weder W. Prospective, randomized comparison of extrapleural versus epidural analgesia for postthoracotomy pain. Ann Thorac Surg. 1998;66(2):367–72. https://doi.org/10.1016/s0003-4975(98)00448-2.
4. Watson DS, Panian S, Kendall V, Maher DP, Peters G. Pain control after thoracotomy: bupivacaine versus lidocaine in continuous extrapleural intercostal nerve blockade. Ann Thorac Surg. 1999;67(3):825–8 . Discussion 828–9. https://doi.org/10.1016/s0003-4975(99)00086-7.

Lobectomies

5

If we were to establish a grading in the difficulty of the lobectomies to be performed and to guide any surgeon who would like to develop a surgical program for thoracic resections of pulmonary malformations, lobectomies are probably easier to perform than anatomical segmentectomies. For lobectomies, resections of "distal" lobes, i.e., lower lobes, are easier than "proximal" lobes, i.e., upper and middle lobes. Indeed, maintaining vascularization and a bronchus for the remaining lobe is more challenging when resecting proximal lobes. Following this grading, extralobar sequestrectomy certainly remains the first intervention to be performed for any surgeon who is a novice in thoracoscopic resections, followed by intralobar sequestrectomy which often requires an atypical resection. Finally, anatomical segmentectomy should probably be reserved for surgeons with some experience in pulmonary resections.

For upper lobectomies, we describe a posterior approach, following an external to medial direction, starting from the first anatomic structure found externally and progressing medially to end up on the vein on both sides.

5.1   Upper Lobectomy

Upper lobectomies are the most difficult to perform for two main reasons:

- An anatomical reason: on the right, starting an upper right lobectomy on the mediastinal side is difficult because the child is in lateral decubitus which hides the mediastinal approach. Furthermore, the right pulmonary artery, which divides rapidly to give rise to the branches for the upper lobe, has a close relationship with the right mainstem bronchus, which makes individualization difficult. On the left, the mediastinal aspect is also difficult at first for the same reasons and the artery is partly hidden by the left upper pulmonary vein.

Supplementary Information The online version contains supplementary material available at [https://doi.org/10.1007/978-3-031-07937-5_5].

- The necessary preservation of vascularization and bronchi for the middle and lower lobe on the right, the lower lobe on the left.

The dissection will most often begin with the section of the inferior pulmonary ligament and this for several reasons: it is most often there that you will find the systemic vessels of a possible sequestration associated with a cystic malformation. It will therefore be necessary to start with the dissection and control of these vessels according to the methods described above. Then at this point we like to initiate the dissection of the lower pulmonary vein and even go around it. This often allows to complete the great fissure in front, starting from the inferior pulmonary vein in order to be sure not to damage it. For this dissection, the grasping forceps placed under the tip of the scapula is helpful to expose the ligament by tilting the lower lobe upwards.

5.1.1   Right Upper Lobectomy (Movies 5.1 and 5.2)

The posterior approach will be described in relation with the particular anatomy described above.

5.1.1.1 Anatomic Findings

On a patient on lateral decubitus, the first anatomic structure we encounter is the main bronchus and the branch for the upper lobe. Just behind will be found the arterial branches. It is the reason why the dissection should be carried on with special care to staying very close to the bronchus in order to avoid the arteries. The number of arteries you will need to control varies from two to three. The first one can even be controlled before the bronchus in the major fissure. For the others, the easiest way is to first control the bronchus and this will open the space, facilitating the identification and dissection of these arteries. At last, the vein will be the last structure to control (Fig. 5.1).

Fig. 5.1 3D lateral view. The fissural artery (posterior ascending artery or apico-dorsal artery) can be controlled first, followed by the bronchus for the upper lobe

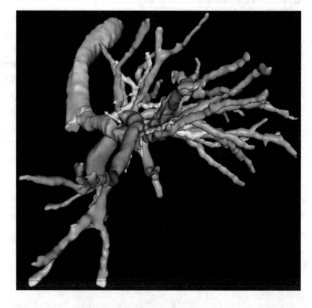

5.1.1.2 First Step: Controlling the Upper Lobe Bronchus

The first step as we said above would be to divide the inferior ligament in order to identify any systemic vascularization for an associated sequestration. That being said, to start a right superior lobectomy by controlling the main right pulmonary artery is difficult in part because the patient is in lateral decubitus making the approach of the mediastinal side difficult and the other part the anatomic location of this artery stretched on the main right bronchus.

On the right side, in a patient in lateral decubitus, the bronchus is outside the artery. Thus, it is simple to start by control the bronchus first before the artery.

As explained above, for a right upper lobectomy, it is easier to start by controlling the bronchus before the artery. The superior lobar bronchus can be found just above the azygos vein. The assistant, using the trocar placed under the tip of the scapula, will expose the bronchus by holding the upper lobe with a grasper. The posterior dissection of the bronchus must be carried out as close as possible to the bronchus, in order to avoid any injury of the mediastinal artery and the branches that will be found once the bronchus is sectioned. For this dissection, either a right angle, a Maryland Ligasure, or a Just-Right 3 mm sealing device can be used.

To control the bronchus, my preference goes towards an absorbable suture (Vicryl 2/0 or 3/0). However, the 5-mm endostapler from JRS offers an even safer control and section of the bronchus, especially in small babies (Figs. 5.2 and 5.3).

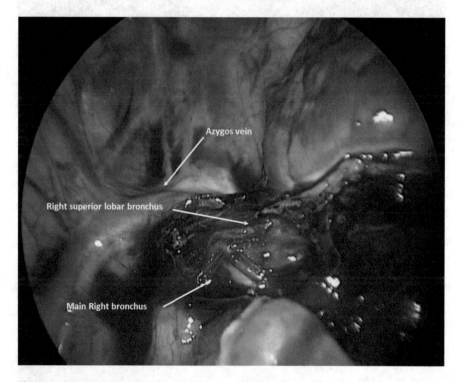

Fig. 5.2 Operative view. The bronchus for the upper lobe is found just under the azygos vein, going up from the main right bronchus

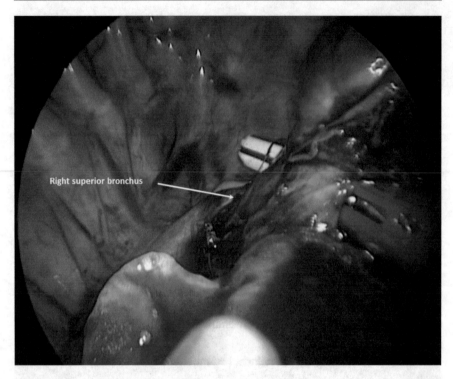

Fig. 5.3 Operative view. The bronchus for the upper lobe has been dissected, with special attention to the mediastinal artery underneath

5.1.1.3 Second Step: Controlling the Fissural Artery (Posterior Ascending Artery, A2)

Once the bronchus has been controlled and sectioned, lifting the bronchial stump up with the left hand allows the dissection of the branch in the fissure, which is the branch for the apico-dorsal segment. There can be up to 3 branches to control, and the dissection should be carried on staying as close as possible to the main right pulmonary artery.

Sometimes, this apico-dorsal branch can be in front of the bronchus and will have to be controlled before the bronchus (Figs. 5.4 and 5.5).

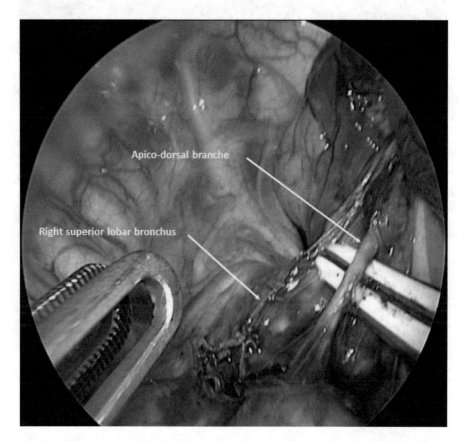

Fig. 5.4 Operative view of the fissural artery (or posterior ascending or apico-dorsal artery), the bronchus for the upper lobe just behind

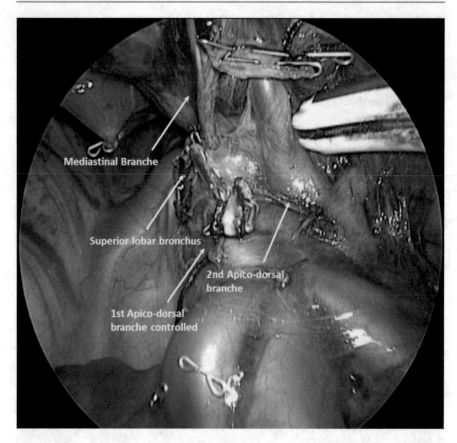

Fig. 5.5 Operative view after control of one of the apico-dorsal branches and the bronchus for the upper lobe, which has been stapled

5.1.1.4 Third Step: Controlling the Mediastinal Arteries (Apical Segmental Artery, A1, and Anterior Segmental Artery, A3)

Once the bronchus has been divided, you will find the two mediastinal arteries. Firstly, the anterior segmental artery which divides into an ascending and a descending branch, and at last, the apical segmental artery that you will control at the end of this arterial step. A sealing device or an absorbable suture can be used to control these arteries (Fig. 5.6).

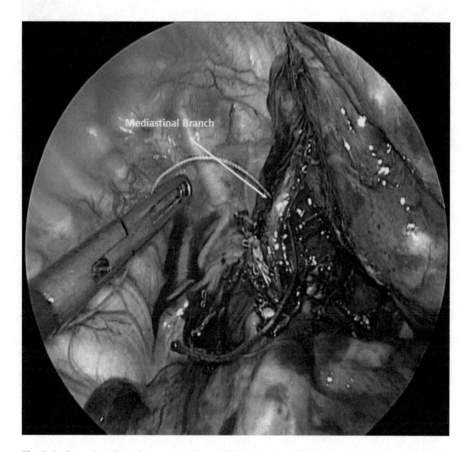

Fig. 5.6 Operative view after control of one of the apico-dorsal branches and the bronchus for the upper lobe (stapled). The mediastinal branch is now ready to be tied. It is not rare to find another branch right after pushing the dissection towards the top

5.1.1.5 Fourth Step: Completing the Minor Fissure

The easiest way is to start from the pulmonary artery that can be found in the fissure. Staying as closed as possible to this artery and carrying out the dissection towards the minor fissure is the best way to avoid any injury of important structures. Care should be taken in order to identify and avoid the artery for the middle lobe, as well as the inferior root of the superior pulmonary vein that drains the middle lobe. A sealing device can be used and allows satisfying aerostasis (Fig. 5.7).

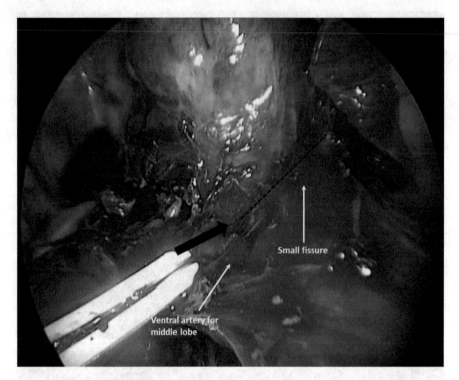

Fig. 5.7 Operative view—dissection of the minor fissure. The black arrow shows the point where the dissection of the minor fissure should be started, once the artery for the middle lobe has been identified

5.1.1.6 Fifth Step: Controlling the Superior Root of the Superior Pulmonary Vein

At this point, the vein and its branches are the only remaining structures to control. I like to make the dissection of the vein as high as possible in the parenchyma so I can use only a sealing device to control all the branches one by one (Fig. 5.8).

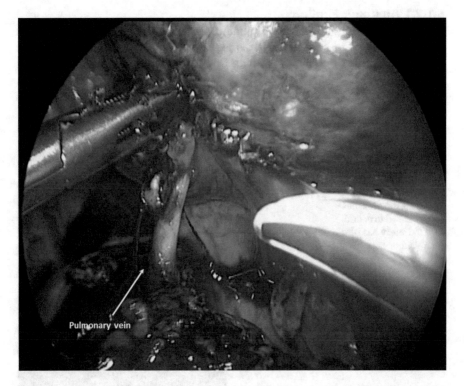

Fig. 5.8 Operative view. The dissection of the minor fissure is completed. The only remaining structure is the right superior pulmonary vein easily identified by lifting the upper right lobe with your left hand

5.1.2 Left Upper Lobectomy (Movies 5.3, 5.4, 5.5, 5.6, 5.7, 5.8, 5.9, 5.10, and 5.11)

As for the right upper lobectomy, the first step is to section the inferior pulmonary ligament.

5.1.2.1 Anatomic Findings

Contrary to the right upper lobe, I found easier to start the lobectomy doing the artery dissection. The lingular artery is the first one to identify because it can start either from the main pulmonary artery or from its basal part which can be a pitfall. In a retrograde direction, the posterior branches should be controlled next. At last, the apical artery (truncus anterior) is tricky to dissect because very high and on the top of the main artery curvature.

Differently to the right lung, the upper branch of the main bronchus will be on the concavity of the pulmonary artery (Fig. 5.9).

Fig. 5.9 3D lateral view.
The yellow dotted arrow
represents the bronchus
you will need to control
once the artery has been
controlled

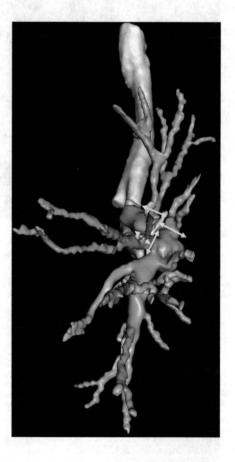

5.1.2.2 First Step: Controlling the Lingular Artery (A4 + 5)

You will find the artery in the fissure. Sometimes, the fissure is complete, facilitating the dissection and identification of the artery. With the patient in right lateral decubitus, the artery is identified more external than medial. A retrograde dissection will be performed in order to identify 3 arteries, from anterior to posterior. You will first have to identify the superior segmental artery of the inferior lobe (segment 6 or Nelson segment) and the basal part of the artery for the inferior lobe. Having done this, you will find the lingular artery, which is the first artery you need to control. The lingular artery can either come from the pulmonary artery itself or from the basal part.

Sometimes, the fissure is incomplete posteriorly. Once you find the plan of the artery, the dissection must be carried on going from the artery to outside in the same plan to complete the fissure.

In case of incomplete fissure, or if the patient has a previous history of infection, it may be challenging to find the artery. The artery may be very deep in the fissure, and inflammatory lymph nodes may make it harder to identify the artery. In this case, a "tip and trick" is to use a stay suture once you find an arterial branch and use a gentle traction to expose the artery and dissect proximally until you find the main artery (see above) (Fig. 5.10).

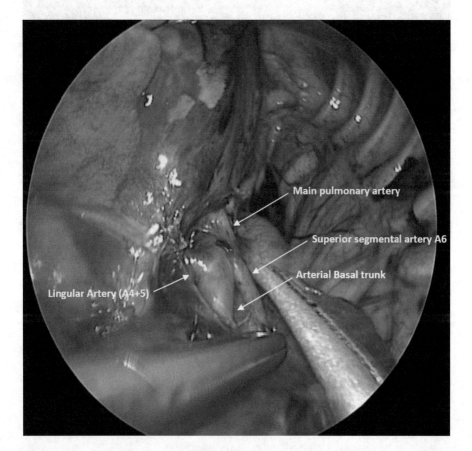

Fig. 5.10 Operative view. The posterior part of the fissure is complete. The lingular artery is easily identified

5.1.2.3 Second Step: Controlling the Posterior Segmental Artery (A2)

The number of these branches can vary from 1 to 3. Immediately after the lingular artery, the posterior segmental artery is the next branch you will find progressing along the inferior pulmonary artery. If the dissection is performed further into the parenchyma you will be able to identify two branches: an ascending branch and a descending one (Fig. 5.11).

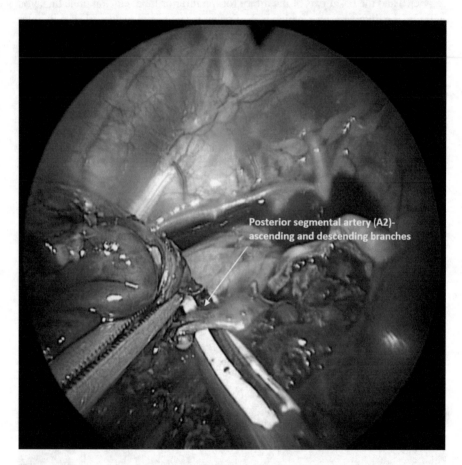

Fig. 5.11 Operative view. Posterior segmental artery identified and dissected right after the lingular artery. At this level you can find two arteries which can be separated and controlled

5.1.2.4 Third Step: Controlling the Truncus Anterior (A1 + 3)

For this dissection, you will need to retract the superior lobe medially using a grasper. This has to be done gently because these segmental branches are very fragile and at risk for dissection, especially in older patients. If you pursue your dissection further into the parenchyma, you will identify two branches from the segmental artery, an ascending and a descending artery. These arteries can be controlled separately or together, depending on how confident you are with the material you are using to control arteries, either the vessel sealer or a stitch. These two branches sometimes have separate origins from the pulmonary artery, which can result in missing a branch that will be controlled at the end of the procedure. At the end of this retrograde dissection, you will have identified the whole inferior pulmonary artery dissected, with all the necessary branches ligated. For reminder, this dissection should be performed as close to the artery as possible, in order to be able to control any potential bleeding (Fig. 5.12).

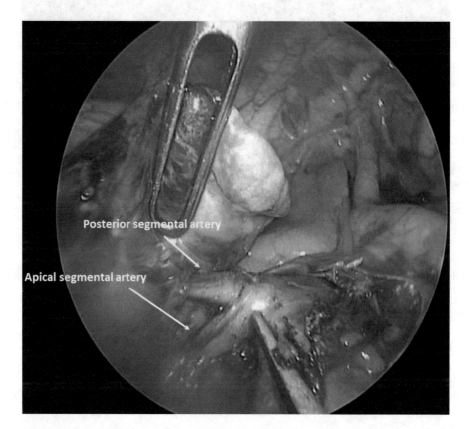

Fig. 5.12 Operative view. The truncus is the last branch to control. Care should be taken with the exposition that is at risk of arterial injury, because of the traction medially. Both branches can be controlled either separately or together depending on the anatomy

5.1.2.5 Fourth Step: Controlling the Upper Lobe Bronchus

Contrary to the right side, the upper lobe bronchus is in the concavity of the artery. You will find it immediately facing the basal part of the artery. At this point, having the assistant grab the upper lobe with the grasper will be helpful to expose the bronchus and both hands of the surgeon free for the dissection. Care should be taken to stay as close as possible to the bronchus posteriorly, in order to avoid injuring the vein that is just behind the bronchus. The bronchus can be controlled either with an absorbable suture or the 5-mm mechanical stapler (Fig. 5.13).

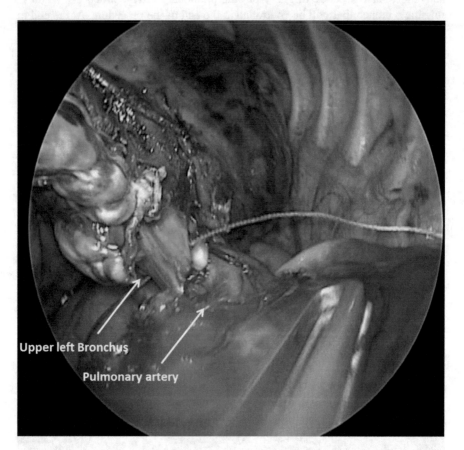

Fig. 5.13 Operative view. The bronchus from the upper lobe is found in the concavity of the artery. As usual, cautious dissection should be carried out, as the vein is just behind

5.1.2.6 Fifth Step: Controlling the Superior Pulmonary Vein

By grasping the lobe towards the top, finishing the dissection should be easy, and the lobectomy will be completed by controlling the vein. The vein may be controlled by a stitch or a mechanical stapler. At this moment, the pitfall is to have a remaining arterial branch that has not been controlled.

Of note, the order between the fourth and the fifth step may be switched (Fig. 5.14).

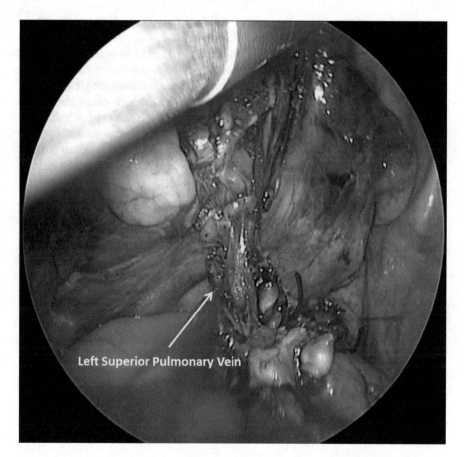

Fig. 5.14 Operative view. The left superior vein is the last structure to control after the bronchus (which is seen sutured in front on the picture)

5.2   **Middle Lobectomy** (Movies 5.12 and 5.13)

Most of the times, the minor fissure will have to be completed in order to do the middle lobectomy. This should be the last step of a middle lobectomy.

5.2.1   Anatomic Findings

In a normal anatomic setting, two arteries will have to be controlled, one lateral and one medial. Often, both arteries share a common trunk that need to be controlled after the vein and the bronchi because immediately behind these two structures. The artery is dissected starting from the arterial "X" in the major fissure formed by the main pulmonary artery, the segmental superior artery for the lower lobe and the basal trunk. The inferior root of the superior pulmonary vein, which drains the middle lobe, will be the first vessel you will need to dissect as it is the most anterior. It is always possible to start by controlling the bronchi, followed by the arteries if you do not want to control the vein first for a drainage matter. However, this makes the procedure more difficult and controlling the vein first is not really an issue (Fig. 5.15).

Fig. 5.15 3D view. The yellow arrow shows the middle bronchus and the others show the arteries you will need to control. You can choose to control these arteries separately or together if they present a common trunk

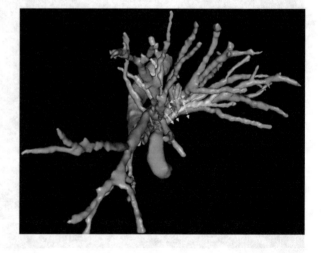

5.2.2   First Step: Controlling the Inferior Root of the Superior Pulmonary Vein

This is the first vascular structure you will find. The dissection is initiated at the confluence between the major and minor fissures in order to find the pulmonary artery. At this point, you will need to identify the basal artery and the artery for the superior segment of the lower lobe (Nelson segment). The inferior root of the superior pulmonary vein for the middle lobe presents two branches for each segment that can be divided and controlled separately. Usually, a vessel sealer alone can be used as these branches are very small (Figs. 5.16 and 5.17).

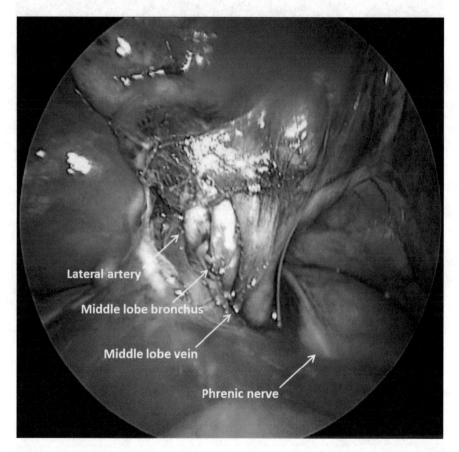

Fig. 5.16 Operative view. After the pleura is opened, this is the anatomic view you need to achieve. As you can see, it will be easier to control first the vein, then the bronchus, and, at last, the artery

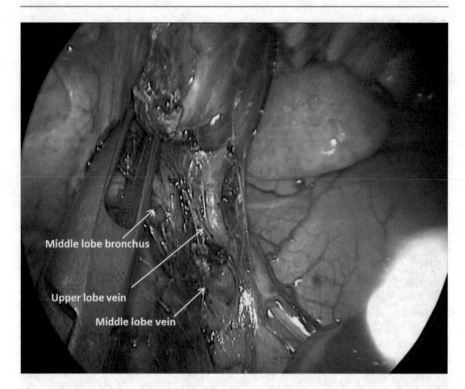

Fig. 5.17 Operative view. The vein for the middle lobe has been controlled and sectioned. On this view, the vein for the upper lobe can be seen and should be carefully avoided when dissecting the vein for the middle lobe

5.2.3   Second Step: The Middle Lobe Bronchus or the Medial Artery

Once the vein has been ligated, the middle lobe bronchus should appear clearly. The dissection should be cautiously carried out, taking care not to injure the lateral artery located just behind. This bronchus is fairly small in a baby and can be controlled by a stitch or a 5-mm mechanical stapler.

Sometimes, one of the two arteries for the middle lobe, the medial arterial, may need to be controlled before the bronchus. Once you will divide it, the bronchus will appear (Fig. 5.18).

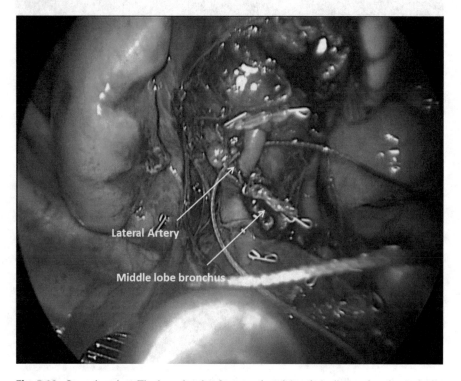

Fig. 5.18 Operative view. The bronchus has been sectioned (stapler), discovering the artery. At this point, you will have only one or two arteries to control

5.2.4   Third Step: Controlling the Lateral Artery

It is the last element to control for a middle lobectomy. Most of the times, the lateral and medial artery originate from a common artery. Sometimes, these two branches can emerge from the pulmonary artery and will be controlled separately (Fig. 5.19).

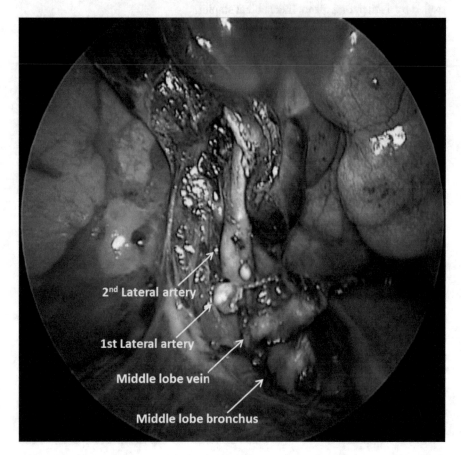

Fig. 5.19 Operative view. In this case, two lateral arteries will be controlled before completing the fissure

5.2.5 Fourth Step: Completing the Fissure

Starting from the artery, you need to find the way to complete the fissure leading the dissection anteriorly. A window should be created, starting from the artery and going towards the mediastinum. Once the window has been created, the parenchyma will be sectioned using either a stapler or a vessel sealer which makes both the aerostasis and the hemostasis (Fig. 5.20).

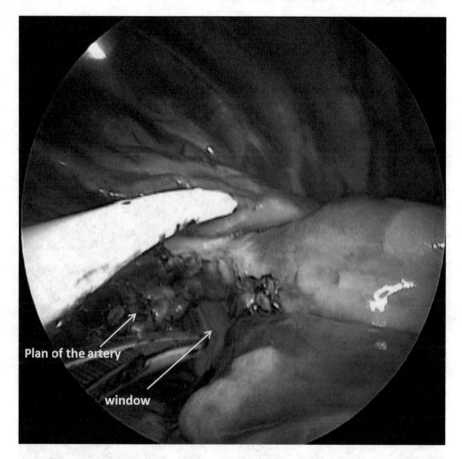

Fig. 5.20 Operative view. All the anatomic elements have been now controlled. Starting from the last artery ligated and staying in front, a window will be created towards the mediastinal side. Once this window is created, the parenchyma can be sectioned

5.2.6   Lower Lobectomy

The lower lobectomy should be the first major thoracoscopic resection a surgeon should perform when starting a thoracoscopy program for CPAM. Indeed, it has the advantage of having a terminal vascularization, only one vein to control (the inferior pulmonary vein), and a terminal bronchial division. The only potential difficulty is having to complete the fissure in the back which may lead to bleeding and missing the anatomy if you are not in the right plan.

5.2.7   Right Lower Lobectomy (Movies 5.14 and 5.15)

As for every lobectomy, the first step should be the dissection of the inferior pulmonary vein and the division of the inferior pulmonary ligament. As mentioned above, this is where potential systemic vessels can be found and controlled (Figs. 5.21 and 5.22).

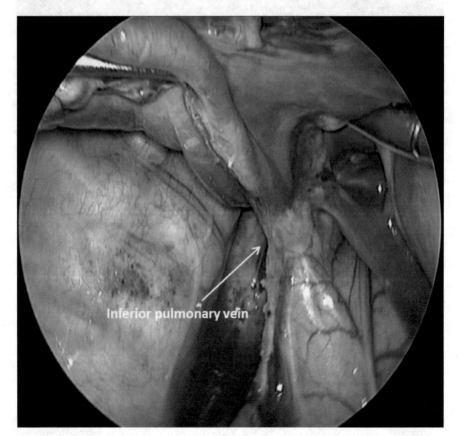

Fig. 5.21 Operative view. The inferior pulmonary ligament has been divided until the inferior pulmonary vein. The dissection of the vein can be initiated at this moment which allows to complete the fissure anteriorly

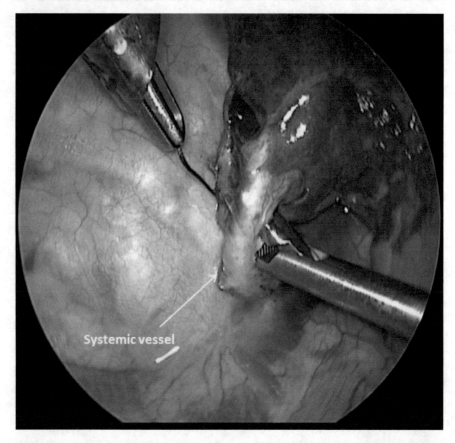

Fig. 5.22 Operative view. Systemic vessels are usually found when dividing the inferior pulmonary ligament. These will be the first vessels to control before beginning any lobectomy

5.2.7.1 First Step: Completing the Fissure

To complete the fissure, the plan immediately anterior to the artery should be found. From there, the dissection should be made laterally in order to create a window. The only structures you may encounter in this plan is interlobar veins that can be coagulated using a Ligasure (Fig. 5.23).

Fig. 5.23 Operative view—completing the fissure. Posteriorly, the artery should first be identified. Once the right plan is found, the dissection should be carried out laterally in order to open a window on the mediastinal side. Any instrument can then be used to cut the parenchyma

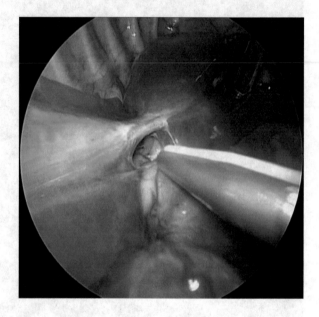

Once the posterior part of the fissure has been completed, you will have to complete the anterior part of the fissure. From here, the basal artery should be dissected, followed by the middle lobe artery and the superior segmental artery further up. This will allow correct visualization of the arterial "X," which is essential in order to avoid sectioning structures that should be preserved (Fig. 5.24).

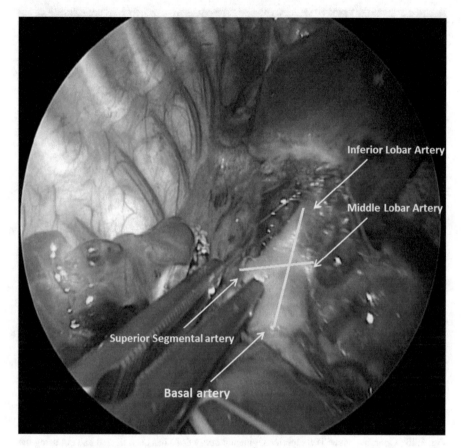

Fig. 5.24 Operative view. This is the view that should be obtained before controlling any artery. The artery for the middle lobe should be perfectly visualized in order to avoid any injury. The arterial "X" is shown in yellow

5.2.7.2 Second Step: Controlling the Superior Segmental Artery

If the arterial dissection has been correctly carried out as described above, controlling the superior segmental artery (Nelson segment) is easily performed using an absorbable suture and vessel sealer (Fig. 5.25).

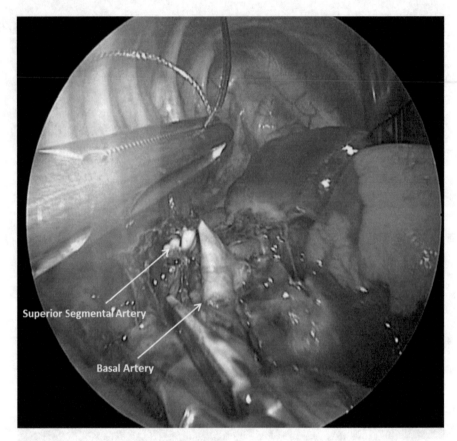

Fig. 5.25 Operative view. The superior segmental artery (A6) has been ligated and cut using the Ligasure. Traction is helpful in dissecting the basal trunk

5.2.7.3 Third Step: Controlling the Basal Artery

Once the superior segmental artery has been cut, and as long as the previous dissection was perfectly carried out, the arterial stump can be grabbed gently in order to complete the dissection of the basal artery. Similarly, a stitch, and/or the vessel sealer, or even a 5-mm stapler can be used for control (Fig. 5.26).

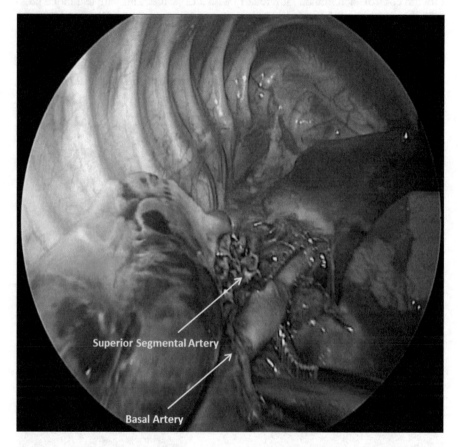

Fig. 5.26 Operative view. The superior segmental artery (A6) is now controlled and sectioned. The next step is to divide the basal trunk

5.2.7.4 Fourth Step: Controlling the Inferior Pulmonary Vein

It is preferable to control the vein before the bronchus. The vein is often very close to the bronchus, leading to a risk of venous injury to the vein during the dissection of the bronchus, especially if there is a history of infection, with inflammatory nodes around. The vein can be dissected as deep as possible in the parenchyma in order to control each branch individually with a Ligasure. This safe technique presents the advantage of leaving a longer stump in case of bleeding, avoiding the retraction of the vein into the pericardium.

A 5-mm stapler can also be used to control the vein, but the stump should still be left long enough in case a bleeding occurs. Before unloading the stapler, the stump should be grabbed with a grasper in order to avoid its retraction (Figs. 5.27 and 5.28).

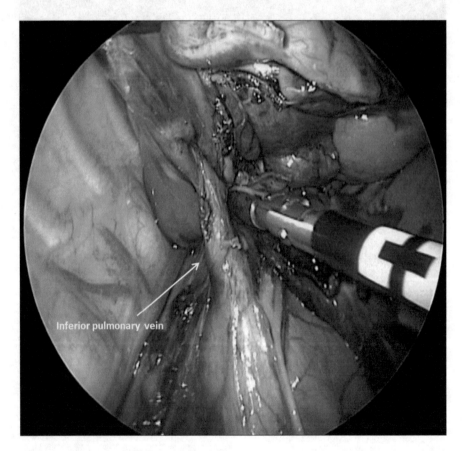

Fig. 5.27 Operative view. The inferior pulmonary vein has been dissected. You can either choose to control each branch individually using the Ligasure, which is safer, or control the whole vein with a knot or using the mechanical stapler

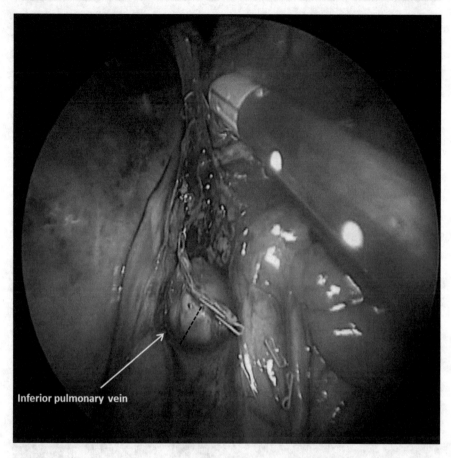

Fig. 5.28 Operative view. The inferior pulmonary vein has been dissected and divided using the mechanical stapler. The stump should be kept as long as possible in case a bleeding occurs. This will avoid the retraction of the stump into the pericardium, which would make the control of a potential bleeding hazardous

5.2.7.5 Fifth Step: Controlling the Bronchus

This is where the surgeon can make a mistake. The bronchus usually follows the same anatomy as the artery, which means that you have to control two bronchi: the one for the superior segmental segment and the other one for the basal segment. The pitfall is to ignore this and control the larger basal bronchus without controlling the small bronchus for the superior segmental segment. This can lead to an air leak which, in the best-case scenario, can be sutured if diagnosed during the surgery, and, in the worst-case scenario, can lead to a broncho-pleural fistula which may take some time to heal spontaneously (Figs. 5.29 and 5.30).

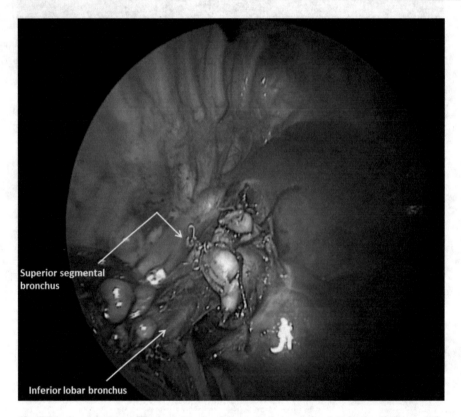

Fig. 5.29 Operative view. The bronchus for the superior segment has been controlled separately from the basal bronchus using the mechanical stapler. A knot can also be used for control

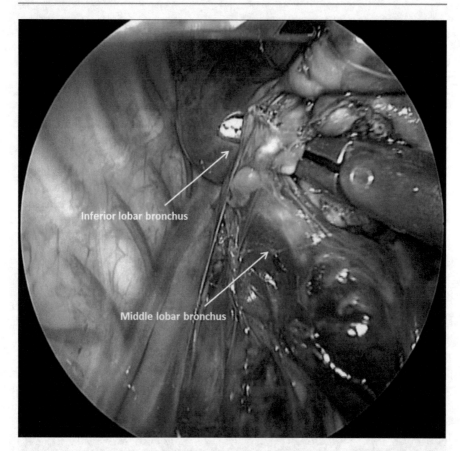

Fig. 5.30 Operative view. Once the bronchus for the superior segment is controlled and sectioned, basal bronchus should be controlled. As you can see on this view, the operator chose to flip the lobe up which can help visualize the bronchus of the middle lobe. You can also choose to keep the lobe aligned to do it

5.2.8 **Left Lower Lobectomy** (Movies 5.16, 5.17, and 5.18)

The procedure mirrors right lower lobectomy. Variations from normal anatomy are more frequent on this side and can include:

1. The lingular artery which can take its origin from the main pulmonary artery immediately above the basal trunk or directly from the basal trunk. This needs to be recognized before controlling the basal trunk to avoid any injury of the lingular artery.
2. The basal trunk can be divided very early in two branches: one for the lateral basal part and a second for the anterior and the medial basal part of the artery. Both can be controlled either separately or together, as long as care is taken not to ligate or shrink the origin of the lingular artery.
3. The anterior lingular artery can sometimes appear rudimentary and should not be taken as a small branch without importance. It needs to be respected (Figs. 5.31, 5.32, 5.33, 5.34, 5.35, 5.36, 5.37, 5.38, 5.39, and 5.40).

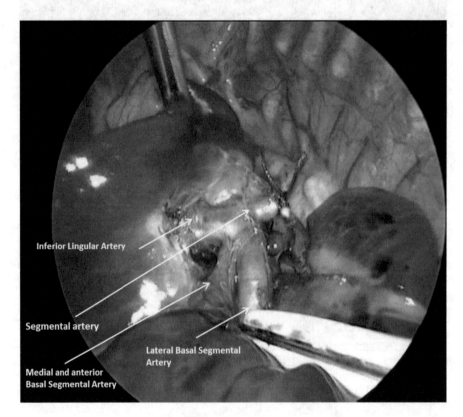

Fig. 5.31 Operative view. The inferior lingular artery is as large as the basal part of the artery. The anterior and medial basal segmental artery needs to be controlled separately from the lateral basal segment

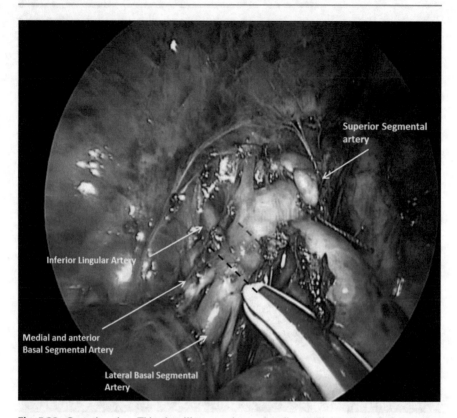

Fig. 5.32 Operative view. This view illustrates the need to dissect all the arteries before cutting any structure. If the dissection is not pushed further, a pitfall would be to control the basal part of the artery following the red line. However, this would interrupt the vascularization of the lingula. Control should be performed following the black line

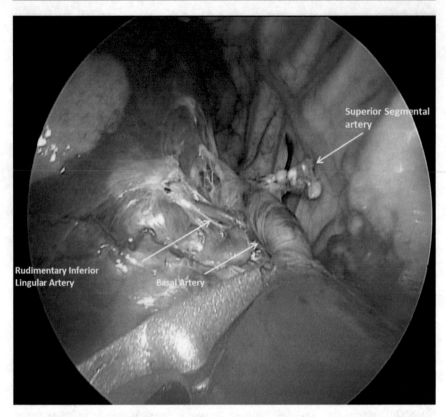

Fig. 5.33 Operative view. On this view, there is a rudimentary lingular artery branch which needs to be preserved. The basal trunk should be controlled distally

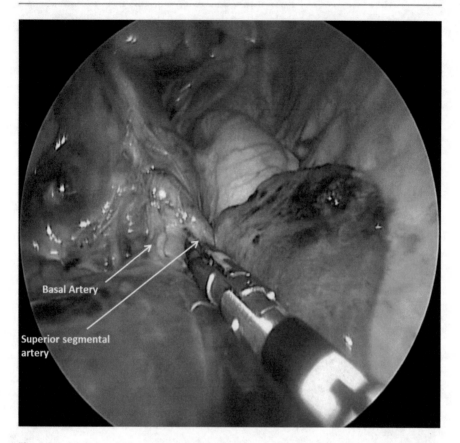

Fig. 5.34 Operative view. As on the right the fissure is complete and the first artery to control is the superior segmental artery (A6)

Fig. 5.35 Operative view. Control of the basal trunk

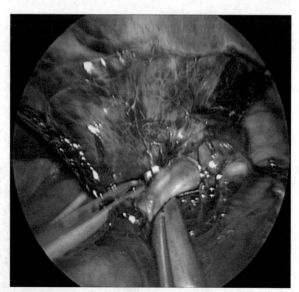

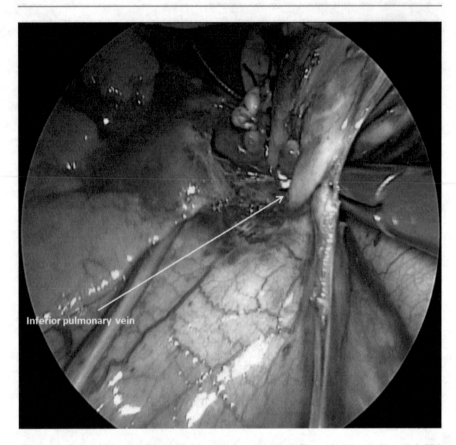

Inferior pulmonary vein

Fig. 5.36 Operative view. The arteries have been controlled. The vein is now dissected. The venous stump should be left long enough to avoid its retraction

Fig. 5.37 Operative view. The vein has been divided using the mechanical stapler

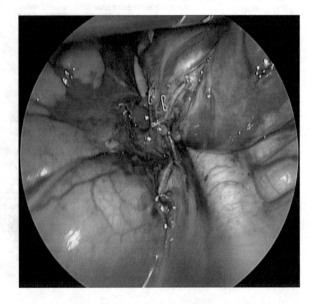

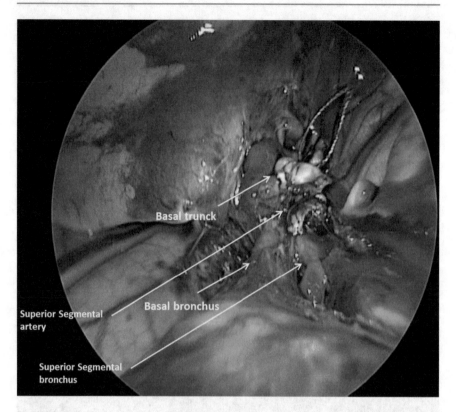

Fig. 5.38 Operative view. The anatomy of the bronchus follows the anatomy of the artery. The bronchus for the superior segment is clearly identified here with the basal part of the bronchus

Fig. 5.39 Operative view. The superior segmental bronchus is controlled here using the mechanical stapler

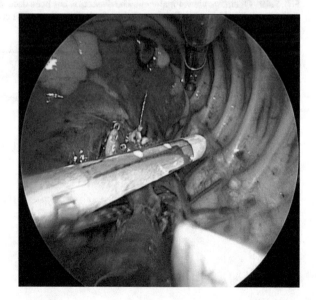

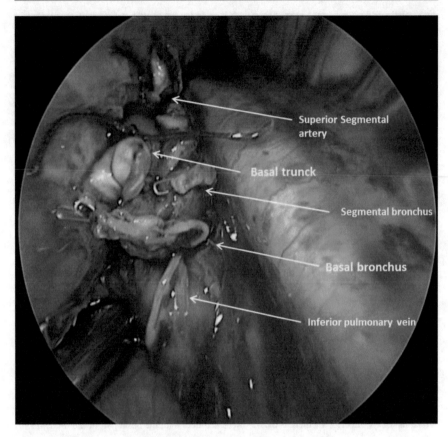

Fig. 5.40 Operative view. Final view. The dissection has been done from the anterior side (artery) to the posterior side (vein). The bronchus is the last structure to be controlled

Further Reading

Gossot D. Atlas of endoscopic major pulmonary resections. Springer; 2018. libgen.lc.

Segmentectomy

6

6.1 Anatomical Segmentectomy

6.1.1 Prerequisite: A 3D Imaging Planner

A comprehensive anatomy of the segment you need to resect is absolutely required. To determine this segment, a 3D imaging is often necessary allowing to localize precisely the lesion, in one segment or multiple segments. In fact, in case of a unique lesion, it is essential to remove all the malformation to avoid any residual disease. As such, a resection of one or even two segments may be necessary. Given the rate of complications after a segmentectomy which appears to be higher compared to a lobectomy, if a resection of more than two segments is required, the surgeon should consider removing the entire lobe instead of leaving in place only one segment, as this would not affect the respiratory status of the child.

In cases of multiple lesions, every effort should be put towards avoiding a complete pneumonectomy. Sometimes, the surgeon will have to be ready to deal with residual disease in this particular case to avoid a respiratory insufficiency related to a major reduction of the parenchyma (Figs. 6.1 and 6.2).

Supplementary Information The online version contains supplementary material available at [https://doi.org/10.1007/978-3-031-07937-5_6].

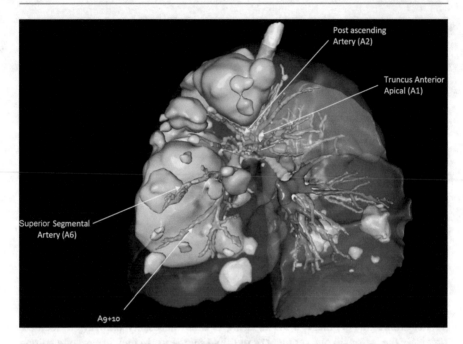

Fig. 6.1 Visible patient application—multiple cystic lesions predominantly in the right lung. By making the image turn around a vertical axis, this application allows to see which artery and bronchus need to be controlled to remove the right segment

Fig. 6.2 Visible patient application—lateral view. Multiple cystic lesions predominantly in the posterior area on the right side. The image has been turned to simulate the lateral view the surgeon will have during the surgery. The segments 7 and 8 for the inferior lobe, the middle lobe (4 + 5), and the segments 1 and 3 for the superior lobe need to be saved

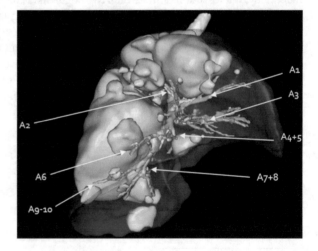

6.1.2   Isolating the Artery with an Antegrade Dissection
(Movie 6.1)

Often, it will be easier to start with the dissection of the main trunk in the great fissure, both on the right and on the left side. A stay stitch is useful to expose the main artery in order to apply a traction and expose the arterial branches further and deeper into the parenchyma. The connective tissue around the artery is divided easily using a gentle traction, similar to the dissection carried out to separate a patent processus vaginalis from the vas and the vessels. As the dissection is carried on further, and depending on which branch needs to be controlled, the stay stitch may have to be moved further to go even deeper into the parenchyma and expose the terminal artery in relation with the segment you want to resect. For control, either a knot or a vessel sealing device may be used (Figs. 6.3, 6.4, 6.5, and 6.6).

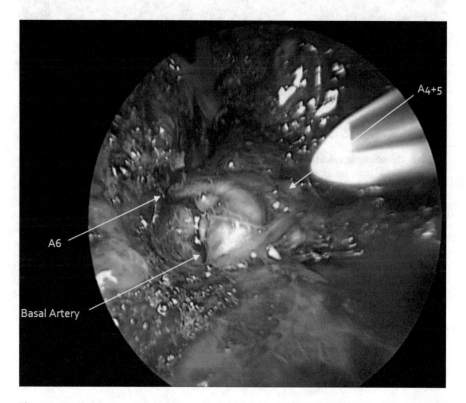

Fig. 6.3 Operative view. This is the same patient presented above with multiple cysts for which a segmentectomy 6, 9, 10 for the lower lobe needs to be performed. The first step is to identify the arteries in the fissure. A6 will be the first to be controlled, followed by A9 and A10

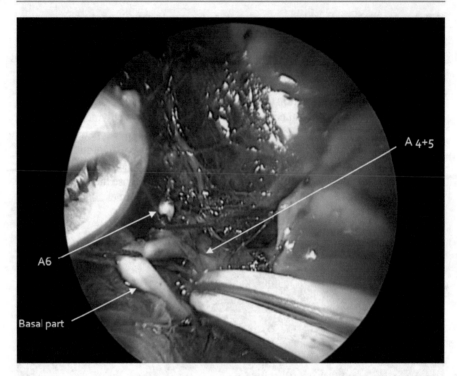

Fig. 6.4 Operative view. A6 has been ligated, and a stay stitch is placed on the common trunk for A9 and A10. This enables the surgeon to identify the arteries going anteriorly in lateral position for the anterior area (A7 and A8)

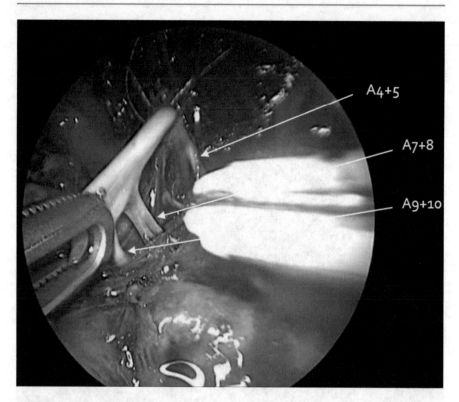

Fig. 6.5 Operative view. A6 has been ligated, a stay stitch is placed on the basal part. The dissection is pushed distally with a traction on the stitch. This way, the surgeon is able to identify the arteries going anteriorly in lateral position for the anterior area (A7 and A8) and A9, A10

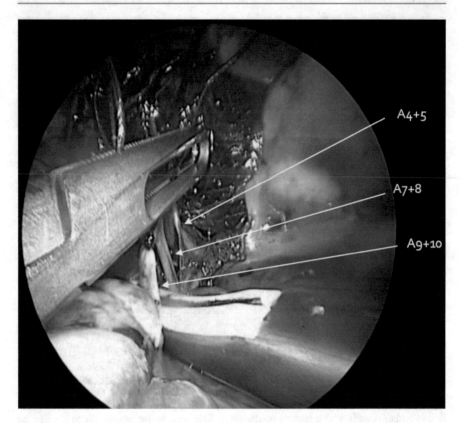

Fig. 6.6 Operative view. A9 and 10 are controlled together using the sealing device which is safe according to the diameter of the arteries

6.1.3 Controlling the Segmental Bronchus

Once the artery has been controlled, you will be able to find the segmental bronchus immediately behind. Using an absorbable stitch, a knot is usually required. Once the artery and the bronchus are divided, an easy way to see where the parenchyma should be sectioned is to stop the CO_2 insufflation allowing the lung to expand and eventually also to ask the anesthesiologist to reventilate the patient. A limit should clearly appear between the segment that needs to be resected and the rest of the parenchyma that will still be vascularized and ventilated. If the cyst is superficial, this also allows to verify that the whole lesion is included in the nonventilated segment that will be resected (Figs. 6.7, 6.8, 6.9, and 6.10).

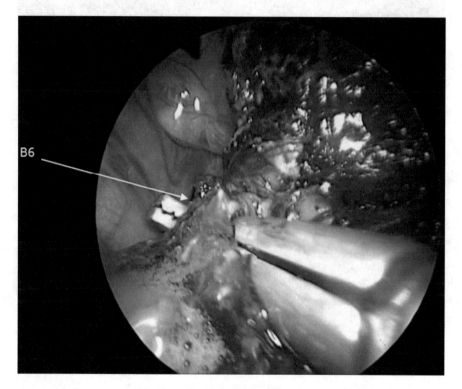

Fig. 6.7 Operative view. The control of B6 is the first step before placing a stay stitch on the basal part of the bronchus. This should be done after the bronchus for the middle lobe has been identified

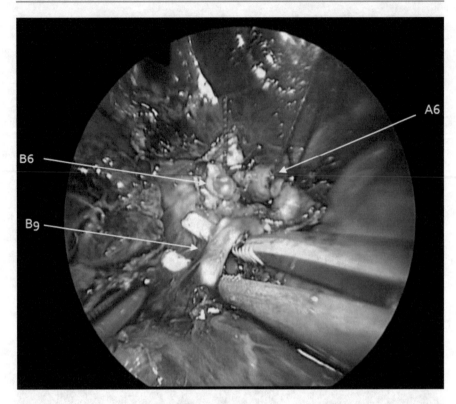

Fig. 6.8 Operative view. By pushing the dissection distally and following the artery with the help of a stay stitch, B9 can be identified and controlled

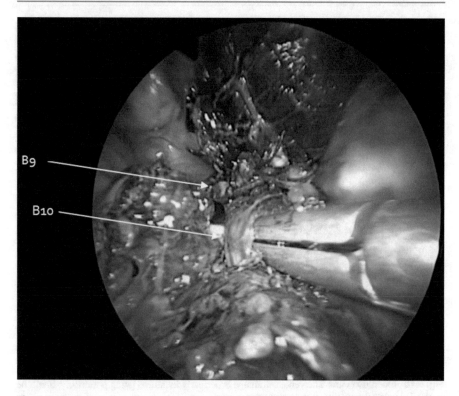

Fig. 6.9 Operative view. The last bronchus, B10, is being controlled, right after B9

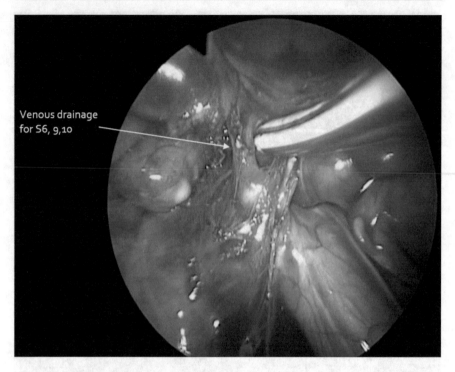

Fig. 6.10 Operative view. The venous drainage is perfectly identified going posteriorly. It will be controlled using the sealing device, or a knot

6.1.4   Sectioning the Vein

Once the arteries and the bronchus have been controlled, it is easier to identify the vein and dissect its branches deep into the parenchyma. This will allow identification in lateral position of the vein that drains the anterior part, which you want to respect in this example, and the branches draining the posterior part, meaning segments 6, 9, and 10.

6.1.5   Sectioning the Parenchyma

Sometimes, sectioning the parenchyma is easier than controlling the segmental vein. Most of the times, the vein is small and will be perfectly divided with the device used to sectioning the parenchyma. A vessel sealing device is very efficient in ensuring the aerostasis and hemostasis for this step (Fig. 6.11).

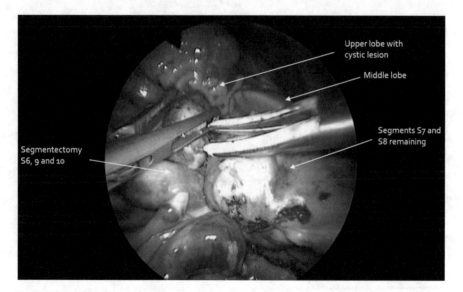

Fig. 6.11 Operative view. The parenchyma is sectioned using a sealing device. The mechanical stapler can also be used. Regarding this patient, a segmentectomy of the upper lobe was also performed

Further Reading

Gossot D. Atlas of endoscopic major pulmonary resections. Springer; 2018. libgen.lc.

Conclusion

This book has been written to help surgeons perform lobectomies in children. It is essential that the surgeon should know the anatomy before considering a pulmonary resection, or, at least, the number and location of the arteries that will be encountered during the dissection. Indeed, it is not necessary to know the name of the arteries, unless for a didactic purpose. Similarly, the surgeon should know how many bronchi will have to be controlled after venous and arterial control.

Dividing the procedure in several steps is crucial to become systematic. Following a step-by-step procedure is the warranty of safety. Similarly, pushing the dissection to identify all the structures is required instead of controlling "en masse" and controlling the vascular structures and parenchyma together. This should be absolutely avoided, as bleeding or a significant air leak will be difficult to fix. No step should be skipped in order to try gaining time. If the order is not respected, i.e., starting to dissect the fissure, followed by the vein, and going back to the artery, and the vein again, etc., it will only make the surgeon lose his/her landmarks, and waste time. Some steps can be inverted but this is not recommended. Usually, the bronchus is deeper in the fissure and controlling the artery first is necessary to access the bronchus. The vein can be controlled first, but might result in venous congestion and hemorrhagic dissection.

And, at last, but not least, do not forget that minimally invasive surgery is an everyday training. Performing a cholecystectomy, a Nissen fundoplication, a splenectomy, and so on is always an occasion to improve your skills knotting, controlling a bleeding, dissecting a vessel, etc. which is something you will need to do to complete a lobectomy. Be confident, you will get better day after day!

Printed in the United States
by Baker & Taylor Publisher Services